IN 3MNT £37.95

£15.00
£10

XX
B

PARALLEL PSYCHOTHERAPY WITH CHILDREN AND PARENTS

PARALLEL PSYCHOTHERAPY WITH CHILDREN AND PARENTS

by
BARBARA PIOVANO, M.D.

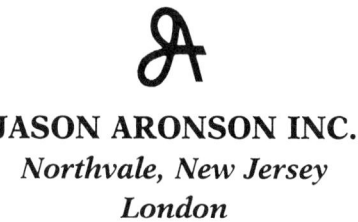

JASON ARONSON INC.
Northvale, New Jersey
London

This book was set in 11 pt. New Aster by Alabama Book Composition of Deatsville, Alabama.

Copyright © 1998 by Jason Aronson Inc.

10 9 8 7 6 5 4 3 2 1

Library of Congress Cataloging-in-Publication Data

Piovano, Barbara.
    [Esperienze parallele. English]
    Parallel psychotherapy with children and parents / by Barbara
Piovano.
       p. cm.
    Includes bibliographical references and index.
    ISBN 0–7657–0126–X (alk. paper)
    1. Child psychotherapy—Parent participation. 2. Parent and
child. 3. Object relations (Psychoanalysis) 4. Child analysis.
5. Family psychotherapy. I. Title.
RJ505.P38P5613 1998
618.92′8914—dc21   97-18427

Printed in the United States of America on acid-free paper. Jason Aronson offers books and cassettes. For information and catalog write to Jason Aronson Inc., 230 Livingston Street, Northvale, New Jersey 07647-1731. Or visit our website: http://www.aronson.com

CONTENTS

CONTENTS

FOREWORD

Barbara Piovano, a skilled and experienced child analyst, proposes that the parents (at least the mother) and the child be treated simultaneously by separate therapists. The therapists would freely communicate with each other and be supervised by the same supervisor. Dr. Piovano discusses this arrangement and several variations in which she might be both a therapist and supervisor.

In the past, these clinical configurations would have been considered a travesty. Even in some circles today, such free and open communications would be viewed as a break of confidentiality leading to a contamination of the transference that inevitably would create unresolvable problems in the transference–countertransference axis. Nevertheless, many of the patients discussed here improved considerably. These patients suffered from severe psychopathology. Some of them were autistic and mute.

Since the second half of this century, psychoanalysis has undergone many changes both technically and theoretically. The emotionally neutral, nonresponsive analyst has become a myth. The therapist is no longer just an analyzing instrument. He is a person with feelings who interacts with patients rather than being a mere reflecting mirror. From a theoretical perspective, instinct theory has become relatively decathected and the role of external objects is being increasingly emphasized.

Whether the patients we see today are significantly different in terms of the severity of psychopathology from those that Freud wrote about is a debatable question. Still, contemporary analysts are aware that we are dealing with severely disturbed patients and that we have to focus on developmental disturbances, especially when treating children. This means that the parent–child relationship is crucial to our understanding of the development and treatment of psychopathology.

Dr. Piovano explores a variety of relationships within the family context simultaneously. I believe her approach is a natural extension of our clinical interest in object relations. The object relations dimension has led to the exploration of countertransference reactions and taught us how they can be useful in the analytic interaction. The object relationship qualities of the analytic interaction once again bring us to the subject of countertransference.

Psychoanalysis is characterized by movements that often become solidified into schools. Once they have reached that level, they claim to represent a new paradigm, to be sui generis, and their antecedents are obscured. For example, it is quite clear that intersubjectivity is a pedantic explosion and description of countertransference interactions that in no way constitutes a novel frame of reference. The same can be said of self psychology, as it is derived from structural and object relations theory which, in turn, are the products of ego psychology. The progression from ego psychology to the study of structural factors and object relations is part of a smooth continuum and a natural extension of psychoanalytic theory that has important implications for the treatment process. Self psychology, instead of acknowledging its use of well known concepts, claims to be a new model.

In the 1950s, I postulated, on the basis of clinical observation, that in long-standing object relations, the character structures and psychopathology of the partners are similar. Particularly in the marital relationship, symbiotic fusion establishes an equilibrium that is adaptive but not necessarily comfortable. Today, those who have turned to the intersubjectivity school speak of codependence, which is a phenomenological degradation of the symbiotic aspects of object relations.

The symbiotic aspects of object relations have to be incorporated in our concepts of psychic development as well as understood in terms of the effects they have on the analytic treatment interaction. It is well known that when a member of a married couple improves because of therapy, the spouse is likely to attempt to sabotage treatment or may decompensate and perhaps seek therapy for himself.

Piovano's attention to parallel process in the treatment of children and their parents is, as mentioned, a natural extension of the object relations perspective and is especially applicable, as a technical innovation, to the treatment interaction. The symbiotic equilibrium of the parental relationship is disturbed or upset because of the child's psychopathology. What had been established on the basis of similarity of character structure can no longer be maintained or be as adaptive as it might have been without the impingements of the child's mental state and behavior. The behavior of the parents relative to each other may have been based on complementarity but derived from fundamentally identical structural configurations such as a sado-masochistic orientation. One partner may assume the sadistic role and the spouse the masochistic, but when events or circumstances interfere with this particular emotional balance, these roles may be reversed or the relationship may collapse, usually because the mother has special ties to her child.

Piovano discusses a variety of ways the mother uses the child for her own needs. The child may not be able to obtain the space he needs to achieve autonomy and to integrate his identity sense. The mother–child relationship may be symbiotic, but not based on equivalence of character structure. If the mother uses the child as an extension of the hated or damaged parts of herself, this may effect a change in her relationship with her husband because now the child is fulfilling and containing certain needs that were expressed overtly or covertly in her symbiotic merger with her husband. The author discusses other types of mother–child interactions and the impact they have on the marriage.

The insights about the different object relations within the family are extremely useful for the individual treatment of family members as well as for the couples therapy that may also be part of the overall treatment program. This book is, in essence, a treatise based on insights gained from the study of family dynamics in a psychoanalytic context, emphasizing an object relations perspective and structural configurations, leaning heavily on the ideas of Melanie Klein and Donald Winnicott. Dr. Piovano also discusses some continental analysts who have made salient contributions, but are not well known in the United States.

Peter L. Giovacchini, M.D.

ACKNOWLEDGMENTS

I would like to express my thanks to Cesare Fieschi, Gian Luigi Lenzi, Massimiliano Prencipe, Camillo Mastropaolo, Giulio Cesare Soavi, Eleonora Fè d'Ostiani, Antonello Correale, Giovanna Goretti, and Roberto Tagliacozzo for their support and trust in advancing the research and clinic project described in the book. I am very grateful to Sergio De Risio for encouraging me to develop, theorize, and write about an experience of many years.

I am indebted to Andreas Giannakoulas, Adriano Giannotti, and Arnaldo Novelletto, who made it possible for me to learn much about children and adolescents and their parents by sharing in the conferences and seminars organized by the University of Rome's Institute of Child Neuropsychiatry.

I would also like to express my appreciation to my supervisees who shared their clinical material with me: Domitilla Cataldi, Silvana Di Vecchia, Nicoletta Lana, Demetrios Rallis, Monica Ricci, Paola Tabarini, and Venanzio Venanzi.

And finally, I owe special thanks to my husband, Siro, for his patience during the writing of this book.

INTRODUCTION

My way of approaching and working with parents in the psychotherapy and analysis of their children has changed over the years. I am referring to methodological shifts from clarification and support psychotherapy to analytically oriented psychotherapy and to more formal treatment of the parents, as well as to my own theoretical transition. The latter entailed a change in my view of parents seeking consultation for their children— not always parents offering adult aspects of the self with which to create and establish a therapeutic alliance in the children's service, no more the "pathogenetic" parents, but parents as people who would never have embarked on treatment for their children, much less for themselves, had not a child's symptoms led them to consult a child psychiatrist. In this sense the child's disturbance offers hope for the child and the parents alike.

My personal as well as my professional growth has favored a change of attitude towards the parents, in that I shifted from a stance of infantile dependency on parental support to one of understanding and cooperation with the parents to the extent of

treating their pathology. While I had to broaden my understanding of the parents' problems and find empathic and collaborative attitudes towards them, my interest gradually extended
from the child to the parent–child relationship and from the
child's disorder to that of the parent. So I tried to establish
favorable conditions (preliminary conversation with parents,
organizing a team of psychotherapists) for offering psychotherapy to parents as well.

The parallel treatment of severely disturbed children and
their parents allowed me to study in depth the influence of real
objects that constitute the current relational context of the child
on his psychic reality, and—vice versa—the effect of the archaic
and pathological functioning of the child on the parent's psyche.
It also gave me the opportunity to intervene in the pathological
interactive aspect of family relationships, while respecting the
setting of both the child's and the parent's therapy. It is common
knowledge that in more serious pathology the intrapsychic
meets the interactive, and individual and family pathology come
together.

The first two chapters are aimed at people who work in
institutions for children and might be interested in following the
difficulties I encountered years ago where I worked as a child
neuropsychiatrist at a second-level center for diagnosis and
psychotherapy of psychic problems in childhood and adolescence.

I first pursued parallel psychotherapy of children and parents in the public service using the methods described in
Chapter 3. The advantage of that setting over private therapy is
that the public service has a staff of several workers. Subsequently, I organized a group of trainee therapists and applied in
private practice the parallel therapy technique that I had developed and theorized in the public service. The idea of offering

one or both parents psychotherapy parallel with that of the child
arose from:

- the need to ensure a stable therapeutic setting for the child
  by removing environmental pressures that have acted and
  continue to act as traumatic factors and that interfere with
  the growth potential gradually revived and released during
  psychotherapy;
- the awareness that a parental request for consultation or
  psychotherapy for a disturbed child often contains a
  denied or as yet unacknowledged request for help from the
  parents themselves, and the consequent wish to provide a
  physical and psychical space for both;
- an interest in exploring family relations, especially the
  narcissistic aspects of the mother–child relationship;
- the need to work on the interactive dimension of family
  pathology while remaining in the psychoanalytic concep-
  tual and technical framework.

The parallel therapy method as set forth in Chapter 4
envisages that: the child and one of the parents (usually the
mother) have parallel psychotherapy in separate settings with
different therapists, the parental couple has regular interviews
with the child's therapist or with a third therapist, the therapists
share some information, and the therapists are supervised
separately by the same supervisor.

The element of supervision of parallel psychotherapies required a model of observation that could embrace the single
therapeutic experience conducted in each setting as well as
bring together and coordinate the work of the therapists. Moreover there was a need to define the field in which the single
supervisor became a participating observer. The field takes its
form from the extended setting that is established after diagnos-

tic assessment and is defined by all the people taking part in the therapeutic experience and their interrelationships. Complex transference and relational dynamics are set in motion between the patient and the therapist, between the therapists themselves, and between the therapists and the supervisor, who thus finds himself at the point of intersection between the anxieties and fantasies of the children, the parents, and the therapists.

Chapter 5 treats a specific theme: aspects of pathological collusion in the mother–child relationship, specifically the narcissistic mother–child relationship. The parallel treatment technique makes it possible to explore the relationship from within the therapeutic relationship of the child and the mother in their respective settings by way of transference and counter-transference as well as through the comparison and discussion of clinical material from the two therapeutic settings. The clinical illustration I have chosen demonstrates the difficulties I had in managing the therapy of a mute autistic child until the mother decided to start a simultaneous therapy in a parallel and separate setting, and the beneficial effects on the child and on his therapeutic relationship produced by the creation of a second setting for the mother.

Chapter 6 considers the theoretical and therapeutic guide-lines and advantages of this technique. I will mention here only two of them, namely the possibility of exploring the unconscious aspects of family relationships and observing how the family is restructured based on intrapsychic changes in single family members engaged in therapy; and the possibility of exploring and taking action on collusions in the mother–child or father–child relationships that interfere with the evolution of the therapeutic process in each setting. Particular attention is paid to the stages through which therapy is articulated at the same time and in the same practice to both mother and child, a simultaneous setting that has proved the most favorable in the therapy of autistic and psychotic children.

Chapter 7 on parallel psychotherapies in psychotic children includes examples that clarify clinical and working hypotheses described in the preceding chapter and illustrates the parallel development of the therapeutic process in the child, the mother, and the parental couple.

In Chapter 8 my aim is to see how far the therapist's thinking and the setting could foster development of symbolization and symbol formation in the psychotic child, independent of environmental changes obtained by involving one or both parents in the parallel setting. Obviously I do not deny the importance of other factors that foster the child's growth, including the therapist's personality (affective availability, patience, tenacity), the receptiveness of the mother and father to even minimal changes in the child, and the contribution of teachers and other people in the supporting environment.

And so to the final chapter. It contains an account of the analysis of a mother who sought consultation for "problems with an adolescent child." In the course of this analysis—the analysis of a patient who would never have sought clinical consultation for herself—an analysis preceded by a long period of preparation, I realized that I had introjected the experience of parallel therapies, those I was directly engaged in and those I supervised, as a model. It allowed me to maintain a wider view of the family and the interactive processes—projective identification, acting out, pathological collusion—that feed the relational pathology and oppose the start and evolution of the therapeutic relationship.

The mother in question, and many like her, have taught me that borderline parents or those with narcissistic personality disorders who come for their children and then start personal treatment are far from considering psychotherapy as an authentic adventure, as a new encounter between two strangers and the occasion for writing a new history among the many possible ones, as Bion would have it (1973, 1978). Instead, they expect the therapeutic experience to be taken home and used to modify family relations that they themselves realize are pathological insofar as they are either dominated by confusional and manipulative narcissistic modes or scleroticized in rigid obligatory paths along which "one person's experience is grafted directly without psychic intermediation on the experience and action of another" (Racamier 1992, p. 140).

As early as the assessment period it is important not to collude with the parental superego in the sense of giving parents tools to reinforce a false self and the control of the child. I suggest instead addressing parents as disturbed or deprived people who are also parents, bearing in mind that they are seeking consultation or therapy not for themselves but for their children.

In psychotherapy it is important at the outset to respect the defensive use that parents make of the child—just as one respects secondary defensive organizations in the patient who comes on his own—until transference is developed and the start of the therapeutic process has dissolved the defensive structures in which the child is enveloped. As for the children, I have learned from psychotic and autistic children that, after all my efforts to meet their needs, I must not forget that they also have desires: the desire to discover the object and the possibility of imagining and dreaming it, the desire to discover the drives and the desire for the object, the desire to change the object and care for it.

1

EXPERIENCES IN CHILD AND ADOLESCENT PSYCHOTHERAPY IN A PUBLIC HEALTH SERVICE

This chapter illustrates the current mandate of the Child Guidance Center I direct with regard to the approach methods and therapeutic proposals relating to psychopathological problems in children and adolescents. The Center, defined as "second level diagnostic and therapeutic service for psychological problems in children and adolescents," treats cases in which alternative solutions, for example, home welfare services, pedagogical and psychological assistance, and other institutions for minors, would be ineffective unless supported by psychotherapy.

For those interested, I have written a historical outline of the structural changes that have taken place at the Center in the last twenty-five years and are linked to the evolution of the Italian social service system. A brief history of the Child Guidance Center in Rome is necessary in order to illustrate the events that determined the present composition of the work group.

The C.G.C. was established early in 1973 as an itinerant psychopedagogical medical team that included a child neuro-psychiatrist (myself), a psychologist, and an educational psychologist. Our specific role was to act as consultants for the Institutions of the Municipal Committee of Rome (institutions that accepted minors assisted by the National Organization for Mothers & Infants [ONMI].)

At the beginning of 1975, the Juvenile Court selected the Center as a consultant agency for couples who wished to adopt children. In the light of this assignment, my collaborators and I asked permission to study, inform, and support the couples during their pre-adoptive entrustment period.

After ONMI was dissolved, in conformity with legislation regarding the decentralization of the administrative, health, and welfare services, we accorded preferential treatment to those institutes located in our district. Since the strictly supervisory work necessary to establish the eligibility of the various institutes was considered incompatible with our personal orientation and professional qualifications, our role became one of permanent consultation.

At this time, we also contacted the work groups directly responsible to the district's administrative agencies (the health and welfare department, the advisory bureau, and the office for the disabled) and the other six C.G.C.s, ex-ONMI, in order to draw up a joint "district-oriented" program.

Generally speaking, over the years the group I coordinate has improved its competence and continues to critically revise its work methods in response to new assignments and the need to remain in close contact with health and welfare services.

The present C.G.C., the last of the seven operational C.G.C.s established in Rome, was created when the itinerant team was assigned permanent headquarters in 1976. The center began to provide child neuropsychiatric outpatient services similar to those of other C.G.C.s, but maintained its own approach methods dictated by previous experience as well as by the professional qualifications and personal orientation of the workers.

The group now numbers three "volunteer" psychologists, two permanent psychologists and myself.

The initial difficulties caused by our integration with the other functioning C.G.C.s were compounded by our difficulties in collaborating with the other health and welfare services which operated in the same administrative district. These included the limited working hours of the staff, problems of coordination due to the slow decentralization of administrative, health, and welfare services, as well as the then current widespread political and ideological resistance towards the need for therapy. *In fact, the one and only solution envisaged was territorial prevention.*

Finally, due to the requests of both users and workers, and based on the proposals put forward during high-level meetings between the representatives of the various district health and welfare services and the aldermen responsible for these services, as well as during municipal meetings, the C.G.C. was defined as a "second level service with diagnostic and therapeutic responsibilities."

As well as other services that fulfilled a preventive role, we repeatedly underlined the fact that the C.G.C. is also effective in global prevention for two reasons; that it contributes to the identification of pathogenic familial and pre-morbid states and that any child therapy is, in fact, preventive with respect to the psychiatric pathology of the adult.

DIAGNOSIS AND THERAPY PROCEDURES

The diagnostic process, conducted with all the necessary technical tools (interviews with children and parents, personality tests, intelligence tests) is, in fact, an extended *therapeutic moment*, because from the very start a relationship is established between doctor and patient.

Instead of directly contacting the prospective clients selected by staff in schools and other health and welfare services, or going to the notifying agency, we prefer to ask the field workers to suggest that the families themselves contact us. This approach seems to fulfill three objectives: to avoid overlapping with other services; to avoid the risk of psychiatrization, whereby direct diagnostic or therapeutic treatment requested by a teacher, for example, might be experienced by the child or family as stigmatizing him and his scholastic career; to test motivation of the parents for treatment. Preference is accorded to those cases that present both more serious pathology and greater motivation.

When speaking on the phone to make the first appointment we try not to influence the way in which the parents requesting the consultation introduce themselves; we let them decide whether to come to the first meeting alone or with the child. This immediately gives us useful information about the person who has the problem (not always the child) and the disturbed relationships that might require our assistance.

I carry out the diagnostic consultation either alone or together with the psychologist who will work with the child and one of the parents. The treatment chosen obviously depends on the diagnosis. The parental couple meets regularly with the child's therapist three or four times a year and, in some cases, also undergoes couples therapy with a couples psychotherapist. This therapy takes place simultaneously with the child's in two adjoining rooms. (In certain situations, and at the start of this work experience, I carried out both the diagnostic consultations and the psychotherapy of either the child or the mother or the parents, as well as supervising the psychotherapists who worked in settings parallel to mine.)

Our initial working hypotheses (later revised on the basis of data acquired through experience, and illustrated in the final discussion) were the following.

- In those cases in which the child presented a minor pathological condition or in which the child's symptoms manifest a personal or family group "maturational" crisis, treatment would be limited to one or two diagnostic-therapeutic interviews with the parents and a certain number of sessions with the child, sometimes with a follow-up and sometimes not; interviews with the teachers, psychologists, and workers who brought up the case, would be held only if they specifically requested them.
- In more structured pathological cases (neurosis, depression, borderline states, psychosis, personality disorders, psychosomatic symptoms) it would be necessary to carry out a psychoanalytically oriented psychotherapy, choosing whether
  - to treat the child with a psychoanalytically oriented psychotherapy if we could establish a sufficiently strong therapeutic alliance during our first contact with the parents, sustained by a small number of follow-up interviews and free of the risk of premature interruption of the child's treatment;
  - to follow the child and one of the parents, or the child and both parents, in separate settings, in those cases in which one or both parents presented an obvious psychopathology or appeared to be so involved that their exclusion would be counterproductive;
  - to propose alternative solutions (more intensive individual psychotherapy or psychoanalysis, family therapy), to be carried out elsewhere, in those cases in which our treatment appeared insufficient.

THE TREATMENT OF ANTONELLA

Antonella and Her Mother

Antonella's mother contacted the Center on the advice of the school's educational psychologist who noted behavioral inhibitions and difficulty in socialization, in addition to a stammer. Mother and daughter came to the first appointment together and were met by me and a voluntary psychologist during a preliminary presentation and data-gathering assessment. The story of Antonella and her family is summarized here with particular reference to the traumas (illnesses and separations) that we believe to be important pathogenic factors in the girl's disorder.

Antonella never spoke, even if she appeared to pay attention and be interested. Two or three times when she did stutteringly try to talk in order to correct or point out something, her mother interrupted, completely invading her space and going on and on about medical data and exams. In the end, Antonella's stammer was presented as the one and only problem.

Antonella's mother is 36 years old. She is the third child in a family from a small town. At present, her family includes a 75-year-old mother who has lived with her ever since an accident in which her own son was driving, and an older brother and sister with whom she is frequently in touch. She moved to Rome when she was 10 and at 12 discovered she had juvenile diabetes; at 23 she lost her father to leukemia and a year later married her present husband. Antonella's father, who is 37 years old and the last of four children, lost his father at the age of 7 and was sent to boarding school until he was 18; he is very attached to his mother and elder sister.

Antonella, an only child, was born one month premature by

a caesarean section due to a maternal diabetic ocular compli-
cation during pregnancy. When she was 1 month old she was
looked after briefly by her grandmother while her mother
underwent surgery for a retinal hemorrhage. At the age of 8
months she was again separated from her mother due to further
hospitalization, this time because of a urinary infection.

Antonella was bottle-fed and had no weaning problems. Her
psychomotor development is listed as normal. She has been
sleeping with her grandmother since she was 3 because she "is
afraid to sleep alone." She began nursery school at 5 and
presently attends fourth grade with a male teacher with whom
she has established a good relationship. She suffers from frequent tracheobronchial inflammations, which were not cured
by the removal of her tonsils at the age of 5.

As it was clear from the start that Antonella's symptom also
catalyzed her mother's strong separation and illness anxieties,
we decided to treat both of them separately, once a week, at the
same time and in adjoining rooms, in order to immediately
establish a *private space* for each. The clinical material illustrated below chronicles and compares the therapies of mother
and daughter. I undertook the psychotherapy of the child and
supervised the mother's; as the child's psychotherapist, I also
met with the parents regularly before the holiday breaks.

Antonella

Antonella is a very pretty, shy, inhibited girl, dressed in an
affected style. Every so often she is shaken by small involuntary
movements. As she says very little and only in response to my
questions, it takes three sessions, complete with drawings and
stimulation figures, to overcome her emotional block. The ice
finally melts after some comments on the drawings, which puts
her into contact with her fear and insecurity. During this first

phase she is unable to express her conflicts verbally, but she makes me strongly feel her sense of impotence and failure when dealing with problems she cannot solve, either by herself or with the help of the family. The diagnostic procedure leads to the hypothesis that, through the use of phobic and counterphobic mechanisms and an exasperated control symptomatically manifest in her stammer, Antonella has tried to provide her own answer to the failure of the primary environment and a solution to her dependency conflict.

Once past the diagnostic phase and certain she will be followed in therapy, Antonella quickly learns to "use" me in order to grow. She produces an incredible series of dreams (told hurriedly and without stammering), and discharges onto me all the emotions and anxieties associated with their contents. She immediately perceives my function to nourish and protect her: this is made clear by certain dreams in which she depicts me as a greengrocer, a butcher, a baker, and her father's boss.

As far back as the first sessions, her dreams portray a small, 5-, 3-, or 1-year-old girl. Each time she comes, thanks to her ability to establish an emotional distance from the various aspects of her infantile self, Antonella is able to talk to me about the impulses, fantasies, and persecutions of "little Antonella" and to bring me, so that I can contain them, her terrible fears of falling, of bleeding, of disintegrating, of dying of hunger and cold. These are the primary anxieties that may be ascribed to the inadequate maternal care and the traumatic separations she suffered during the first months of her life.

When one of her goldfish dies Antonella tells me the following dream: "I kept this dead fish in a box and didn't throw it away until his eye deflated (the mother suffers from diabetic retinopathy and has very poor sight). . . . The other fish was fine." She then associates: "the remaining fish is one year old on March 15th, my mother's name day is March 16th, and my birthday is March 17th. In my dream," she continues, "the other fish also dies." I contain her present death anxieties for her mother and herself, which are revealed in her dreams, by telling her that she is re-experiencing a fear and terror she had felt (in the sense of "fear of breakdown," Winnicott 1974) when she was so small that she couldn't cope, and that now she can stop worrying because her mother is being treated by good doctors, is fine, and can take care of herself and of Antonella.

The Mother

The mother appears as a classically dressed, well-groomed young woman, whose expression and attitude betray the belief that attack is the best form of defense. That is, every attempt at the beginning to make her contact her feelings, emotions, or needs creates a context in which she can recognize herself as a patient; she rejects such attempts as persecutory ("I'll solve my problems myself. If it weren't for Antonella I wouldn't be here"). Her extremely defensive and sometimes negativistic attitude does not stop her from coming regularly to the sessions; her mood swings range from more frequent manic states to depressive ones.

Her explicit demands for advice and approval and the way she tries to include everything in her sphere of omnipotence, even if this means "taking the blame for any faults and accepting total responsibility," betray a strong need for dependency and totally denied aspects of fragility of the self. The needy infantile self of the mother is projected onto the daughter: the mother also seems to have overdeveloped a hyperprotective maternal attitude of a "false self" type. Mother and daughter have not individualized and differentiated from one another. Even some of the contents of the mother's phobias are the same as her daughter's: oxen, dogs, mice, and thieves. Like the daughter, the mother was always afraid of sleeping alone and passed from her parents' bed to that of her husband. Both present similar experiences regarding the fear of falling, being ill and dying, and both tend towards somatic reactions to separation (colds, fever, colitis).

One easily understands how Antonella's mother, so centered on her own needs and with such conflictual and traumatic past experiences, could have failed to fulfill her function of *holding* and *reverie*. Subsequently, through mechanisms of reciprocal projective identification between mother and daughter, a vicious circle began at a level of unconscious communication, and this slowed down the separation-individuation process, increasing a confusion of their identities and building a *disturbed relationship*.

The separate treatment of Antonella and her mother and the creation of their own "private space" were aimed at breaking this vicious circle and fostering the acquisition of separate identities. This produced an imbalance in their relationship with a tendency towards acting out as well as swings between regression and escape in the growth of both mother and daughter. When Antonella's search for new objects (friends, father) and for independence was at its strongest, the mother became "empty" and "depressed," and reacted by developing a number of interests that led her to associate with her nieces and nephews. The mother's new contacts in turn provoked feelings of jealousy and abandonment in Antonella, which her therapist had to repair. After the mother missed two sessions, Antonella invented or hallucinated a telephone call from her therapist to her mother intended as a reprimand, and on another occasion, enacted a fantasy of omnipotent control by involving her father.

Of the two, Antonella seems the more motivated towards therapy; the mother, while clinging to the therapist, continues to resist the analytic work. A tentative prognosis seems more favorable to Antonella due to her strong vitality and desire for growth; promoting a change in the mother is altogether a more difficult and delicate task. Antonella's therapy will center on anxiety containment and facilitation of her insight, as well as on reinforcement of both the ego functions and the more ego-syntonic defense traits.

THE TREATMENT OF RAFFAELE

Raffaele and His Mother

Mother and son come together to the first appointment and are received by me and the therapist who will treat the son.

The mother draws a desperate picture: "Your name was given to me by X, but it's no use. Raffaele refuses to study. As soon as he starts something he loses interest. At school he's a disaster. He still can't write, and I had to drag him here. He's always like this." As if echoing his mother's words, Raffaele walks towards the door to leave but his mother stops him with a crippling look saying: "There, you see!" She continues by reeling off a long list of medical data, obviously learnt by heart, and only when she starts to talk about herself and her family does she begin to show any emotions. I become the mother's referent. Raffaele no longer exists; he's crumpled up on the chair and his mother seems to remember he's there only when she tells me, winking in a confidential manner, "things he really shouldn't hear."

The mother is a firstborn child who has worked since she was 14. She married a first cousin at 27, the year her mother died. At the time, her father was about to marry his dead wife's sister, "a typical warmonger" who had been forcibly introduced into the household by a wealthy relative and had been having a relationship with the father for some time. During the honeymoon "my suitcases were stolen and immediately afterwards my husband lost his job." By telling me about these two events she communicates not only her disappointment that her marriage fell short of her expectations, but also how she felt robbed of all the privileges she had enjoyed in her own family while her sister had been burdened with responsibilities at an early age. She lived with her in-laws for the first eight months of her marriage; her husband finally found a steady job four years later.

Raffaele, the second son, was an unwanted child. It was the guilt she felt for this initial "refusal" that prompted her to give him "much greater affection." Breast-fed for a month, then bottle-fed, he had no weaning problems and always had a voracious appetite. Between the ages of 2 months and 2 years he was looked after by a young woman who let him sleep during the day so that at night he had nightmares and constantly sought contact with his mother. He had several phobias, including the rubber gloves used by the woman mentioned above. His psychomotor growth was delayed, language in particular; a number of medical exams ruled out organic causes. When beginning nursery school he had repeated bouts of vomiting. Apart from his brother, he refused to stay with other boys because he was afraid of being attacked. The mother slept with Raffaele until he was 5, while the father slept in the parents' bed with the older son. The wife describes her husband as a reserved, introspective man who considers his family as a "chain around his neck" and when at home is "only a body," so that everything weighs on her shoulders. Raffaele presently attends fifth grade and is scholastically "so behind" that the mother thinks he should repeat the academic year. The consultation therefore becomes a sort of request by the mother for authorization to leave her son in fifth grade so as to avoid the anxieties caused by his advancement to high school.

Raffaele's second diagnostic interview takes place alone with me. He refuses to come in, runs away, shouts insults, and only when I tell him that perhaps he is afraid to come in and confide in me lest I abandon him as other doctors did in the past does he finally agree to sit down and draw. He does some drawings by himself (a raindrop that breaks off from a cloud and falls into a river, a storm in which his father with an umbrella calms his son, a rocket with a person inside who says "hurrah, I'm going to the moon") as well as others whose theme I suggest (anger—a muscular man, the home—mother and son, some of which he draws and some he makes me draw, dictating the words I have to write in the balloons to make the people talk. Through the drawings he clearly indicates that he is immersed in an extremely fusional and ambivalent relationship with his mother and cannot count on his father or brother to break away.

During the third and last diagnostic interview I meet both parents: the father confirms the picture painted by his wife, of a person reluctant to consider problems from a psychological point of view and generally unwilling to converse. Frustrated in his attempts to teach Raffaele, he believes him to be retarded and spoiled by his mother. The wife constantly seeks my support in an attempt to make her husband more open towards their son, at the same time disqualifying and assailing him about his job and all the activities he considers as his hobbies. At the end of the diagnostic consultation I propose a parallel psychotherapy to mother and son, in the hope that any future change will impact on the rest of the family.

The accounts that follow describe the mother and son's therapies and aim at highlighting the changes in the two therapeutic relationships. I undertook the mother's therapy while the son's was carried out by a psychologist under my supervision. The son's therapist was readily available to meet the parental couple on a regular basis: the father, however, never showed up.

Raffaele

Raffaele is a sturdy, chubby, 12-year-old boy with brown hair. His movements and expression are somewhat ungracious and he has a shifty yet sharp and penetrating gaze. From the very first session he manifests delusional aspects (fear of being poisoned with medicines, of being ridiculed), omnipotent defenses, and denial of any form of weakness, as well as autistic-type defenses (when he tells about a dog preserved on ice I think he refers to his infantile self), which prevent an emotional contact with the therapist. He refuses to enter the room when he feels it to be contaminated by the projection of internal sadistic and persecutory objects, and violent, aggressive, or "mad" aspects of self. Not always does interpretation reduce the feelings of persecution, so for much of the hour both therapist and child remain outside the room. By telling a story of Sandokan (an Italian adventure hero) in which a woman saves him from the enemy but at the same time condemns him because she puts him in a sack, Raffaele communicates his conflict: his inability to separate from his mother, who he continually fears will engulf him. Before analytic breaks, he brings various objects from home, a small rocket and a magnet; he plays with them to express his adhesive relationship with his mother and his terror of being catapulted into space. Every time he contacts the need and anger he feels towards his mother and the therapist he attacks therapy dependency, discredits the therapist, and escapes into self-sufficient fantasies ("everyone's shit, I don't need anyone"). He repeatedly acts out his aggressiveness by bringing scissors, belts, and guns from home and points them at the therapist.

During the subsequent phase, the clinical material shows splitting defenses between good and bad objects (cops and robbers, the police protecting a bank), and attempts at integration of the self (he draws an engine with pistons and cylinders that work together) and at reparation of the object (he gives the therapist a pen holder, but throws it on the floor as soon as he compares it to the therapist's). Once again, the time comes to leave primary school and move on to high school: on this occasion, the mother, while in the other room, tells of certain dreams in which she can no longer find Raffaele and tearfully relives her own departure from primary school. Raffaele tells his therapist of his own sense of inadequacy and inability, of his lack of confidence in a future job, of his regret—immediately denied—at having to leave his female teacher. On a deeper level all this is experienced as falling into a gorge and being poisoned.

At the end of the first year of high school, the improvement in his behavior (he does not let his mother dress him, he goes to the swimming pool, accepts tutoring from a boy, and tries to make the therapist jealous) appears to be the result of secondary identification with the male therapist, his father, elder brother, and uncle.

The Mother

Stout, with a decisive and efficient air about her, she reveals a rigid character structure that does in fact function in a large area of the ego. I am able to involve her by presenting myself as at once her son's co-therapist and her own auxiliary ego. In the first case, we are working together to identify the anxieties and conflicts at the root of her son's behavior; I repeatedly explain his aggressive attitude and negativism (which exasperate her most) as his need to differentiate himself from her, and attribute his extreme voracity to an intense need for protection and affection. In the second case, the task is to help her recognize in her son her own fragile, dependent, hungry, and rejected self, and to contain both her son (*instead of containing she has always "explained" to her son*) and the threatening parts of her own internal world that he enacts (*"He actually does what I dream*: escapes, argues," and so on).

She gradually becomes the patient. I am able to bring her into contact with the emptiness she feels every time her son moves away (which she tries to fill with a thousand other things) and with her own aggressiveness and rivalry with her parents, her mother-in-law, and, above all, her husband. Her extremely incoherent attitude towards her son's destructiveness demonstrates how his aggressiveness was fusionally used to maintain an intrapsychic balance and also as a protest against her husband and the environment.

Raffaele's pathology appears to depend on a distortion of the mother–son relationship during the separation-individuation phase: a mother with an insufficient sense of self who uses a son as an integrating part of her own self and keeps him in a state of fusion, a child who feels invaded by his mother's personality and cannot reach (due to personal traits) sufficient levels of integration to allow him an undistorted relation with reality. Both of them felt the therapy to be an opportunity to experience an emotional relationship as well as a possibility to broaden their field of experience. Even if frustrated and full of hate due to having been caught in a vicious circle of sterile and defensive thinking with no way out, the mother is, however, a lively and sensitive person who, apart from her rigid defense mechanisms, is open to anything she feels is "good." Raffaele does not hate reality, but rather the only reality he has ever known—a *pseudo-reality of symbiotic origin* (Searles 1974), from which he attempts to emerge with a healthy aggressiveness, even if apparently sadistic, castrating, and destructive.

DISCUSSION

The foregoing case histories stress that only a small number of subjects assessed requested our assistance for organic pathologies even though the C.G.C. is generically categorized as a second level diagnostic and therapeutic service for neurological and psychological problems in children and adolescents. In fact, in the last few years, the clients have shifted from being subjects with neuropathological problems to those with psycho-affective and relational disorders.

I believe that this change in clients is determined by three factors: self-selection by the clients who exclude organic causes through prior medical examinations, greater awareness of the local service workers regarding psycho-affective and relational disorders, less resistance towards mental illnesses—this can be considered as a greater capacity to identify conflictual and relational situations as the cause of psychophysical discomfort.

The specific experiment my collaborators and I conducted is based on introducing a number of observations, operative concepts, and psychoanalytical theories into the field of infantile psychiatry carried out in a public service. This has proved to be useful as a research method, as a propaedeutic and collateral activity to psychoanalytic training (in the sense that it favors the psychotherapeutic potential of those who have just begun psychoanalysis), and also as a therapeutic method. Even though I agree that psychoanalysis as a therapeutic method requires too much time and energy to be provided on a widespread basis, the number of cases in which we have been able to carry out psychoanalytically oriented psychotherapy has been propor-

tionally sufficient with respect to the demand, due to the
introduction of certain changes in the technical psychoanalytical model. These changes left the fundamental parameters of
setting and *motivation* intact while adapting to the particulars
of the work environment. First, organizational difficulties and
time constraints made it impossible to spend more than one
hour per week with each person; we did, however, avoid changes
in the timetable and guaranteed that no other patient would be
received during each appointment hour. Second, as therapy was
free, motivation was not guaranteed by the economic factor; it
was tested from the start by means of a series of conditions that
the users had to *actively* overcome in order to benefit. (Free
treatment conjured up various fantasies, some of which were
commonplace ["second rate" therapy], while others were more
specifically situational and were examined case by case.)

We tried not to fuel excessive expectations on the part of the
parents as to the likelihood of their receiving practical assistance, for instance, with applications for unemployment benefits or direct involvement with the school board. We sought to
counter infantile dependency with more adult and collaborative
traits, or involutive and destructive attitudes with vital and
constructive ones.

The therapeutic factor was identified in emotional-cognitive-
relational growth and maturation. This is in contrast to the
more diffuse and deep-rooted traditional medical model, which
considers the "damage to be repaired" as the doctor's therapeutic task while the patient plays only a passive role. This viewpoint is based on the way we approached each patient and
developed the relationship. What proved to be utopian was our
initial hypotheses that we could carry out individual psychotherapy with the child and limit work with the parents to a
certain number of interviews aimed at establishing and maintaining a therapeutic alliance. Despite the time limits and the

reductive changes mentioned earlier, I came to recognize the advantage of a public service in cases of child and adolescent psychopathology as an institution with a number of working psychotherapists, as against a private practice with just one. The fact that we were a group actually permitted us to carry out separate initial diagnostic studies on the intrapsychic structure of the single patient and on interactive couple and family dynamics. Subsequently, we were able to involve more than one family member in separate treatment. This technique facilitates a wider range of interventions, including: carrying out simultaneous treatments, thereby saving time; acting earlier (than private practitioners can) in those situations in which parents are still unable to recognize themselves as patients and, therefore, cannot initiate their own therapy unless they find a service that considers their involvement in the treatment routine; effecting a real but not excessively traumatic separation by carrying out simultaneous sessions in adjoining rooms in cases of mother–child symbiosis (like Raffaele's).

The cases in which we obtained our best results in a relatively short space of time are precisely those involving distortions of the early mother–child relationship, with a pathology in both the child and the mother (Giannotti and De Astis 1981). Even if we often observed a psychopathology of the father (or other family members, for example the grandmother) and father–son relational disorders, we worked mainly with children and their mothers since they were the ones who were in fact more available during the open hours of the Center. From a social point of view, we noticed that the whole family tended to use this outpatient facility; this seemed to us a reassuring confirmation that the public health service is currently not considered simply a place in which to "offload" the problem child.

2

PSYCHOPEDAGOGICAL TREATMENT AND PSYCHOANALYTICALLY ORIENTED PSYCHOTHERAPY

INTRODUCTION

This chapter further documents the work of a Child Guidance Center in one of the District Health Services of Rome, part of the National Health Service program that envisages and encourages collaboration and coordination between district welfare and health services. We have already discussed the methodology used in diagnosis and choice of treatment, illustrated the treatment—psychoanalytically oriented psychotherapy—with two clinical cases, and hypothesized that the change from subjects with neurological problems to those with psychoaffective and relational problems could be attributed to the efficiency of the local services in the District, among other factors. I now wish to stress the role of one of the local services—the school operators—in identifying the psychological problem of a child or family and in motivating the family to use psychotherapy in order to deal with it. In particular, I wish to underline the importance of the figure and role of the educational psychologist in recognizing a

psychopathogenic risk situation on the basis of a psychopedagogical evaluation, which requires further clinical assessment
and possible psychotherapy.

Three clinical cases are described in this chapter. Two were
initially treated at length in the school and only later came to the
C.G.C.; the third was followed from the start by therapists at
the Center, which was contacted directly by the parents because
of the son's difficulties during his first year at school. Positive changes were recorded and examined jointly from time to
time by the school operators and the psychotherapists working
at the Center. This prompted me to try to identify the criteria
that distinguished analytic psychotherapy, and specifically the
Center's parallel psychotherapy of parents and children, from
the psychopedagogical and broadly defined psychotherapeutic
treatment already available in schools.

The last part of the chapter stresses the importance of the
school as a social environment either complementary and/or
alternative to the family, and its preventive role in pinpointing
and identifying, early on, a psychopathological risk situation.
The advantages and disadvantages of motivation deriving from
the school rather than coming spontaneously from the family
will be discussed through the comparison of the clinical cases.
Finally, we consider if and when the cases reported by the school
would have otherwise sought psychotherapy in either a public
health service or in private practice.

NORMATIVE AND FORMATIVE CHANGES IN SCHOOLS

The implementation of legislation regarding the introduction
into regular schools of children with physical and psychological
problems was met with a variety of reactions in scholastic
circles. Initially there was a refusal of the disturbed child owing

to the teacher's lack of specific training and to difficulties in updating traditional teaching methods. Subsequently, after the introduction of such new staff members as a school psychologist and an educational psychologist, there was a tendency to hyperprotect the child and an argumentative attitude towards parents and teachers stemming from excessive identification with the child or a hypercompensatory defensive attitude towards him. Finally, there was an improvement in the skills of school workers who, without using medical instruments, were able to make an initial macroscopic distinction between "mental insufficiency of organic origin" and emotional and conflictual learning difficulties; an increased psychological sensitivity in interpreting the factors that favor or hinder the formative educational process; and an increased commitment to proposing and implementing specific interventions in response to a variety of personal, scholastic, and social problems.

THE EDUCATIONAL PSYCHOLOGIST AND THE IDENTIFICATION OF A PSYCHOPATHOLOGICAL RISK SITUATION

The educational psychologist who assisted in the preparation of this chapter has drawn on his school experience to define his role, propose an operative technical model for research and work, and indicate the criteria that denote a psychopathological risk situation requiring clinical assessment. According to the Ministry of Education, he is the "teacher expert in educational psychology": his role is to integrate the work of the other teachers and coordinate local workers both inside and outside the school; it differs from that of a clinical psychologist or a psychotherapist. When dealing with the various problems inherent in school life (cases of maladjustments and scholastic delay, inclusion of pupils with disabilities, family problems interfering with education, relationship difficulties between school workers and pupils), the educational psychologist prizes the prevention and cure of a pupil's psychic discomfort as the sine qua non for a normal learning and socialization process. He divides his work into two phases, cognitive and operative.

During the cognitive phase he begins by systematically observing, in the classroom, the children reported by the teacher; he then interviews the child and his parents. Finally, using a series of technical research tools chosen case by case, he evaluates development in the various ares of personality and formulates a psychopedagogical diagnostic profile for each child.[1]

During the operative phase, while teachers are adopting specific learning techniques to increase the child's cognitive development, the educational psychologist establishes a trusting relationship with the child by putting him in contact with his emotional difficulties and needs, and focuses on promoting development of the self by using expressive activities (either one-on-one or in groups), and facilitating the child's relationship with his teachers and peers. At the same time, he conducts systematic and repeated interviews with the mother or with both parents to make them aware of the child's difficulties and involve them emotionally in the search for a solution.

When the work described above, together with any medical

---

1. The diagnostic tools most often used individually were family history, tests/exercises that explore the dynamic framework of the pupil's psycho-social maturation, visual perception tests (Frostig), language tests (Frostig), Vajer's psychological test, intelligence tests of cognitive learning, exercises to detect and assess dyslexia, drawing of human figures, drawing of the family, pupil interviews. Tools most often used in the class setting were Moreno's sociometric test, free drawing and the invention of fairy tales to express fantasies, experiences, and desires, Flanders analysis of teacher–child interaction, psychodrama, music.

treatment carried out by school doctor, pediatrician, or neuro-psychiatrist, is not sufficient to alleviate the disorders that interfere with the normal affective-cognitive-relational develop-ment of the child, the educational psychologist attributes the persistence of psychic discomfort to either a neurotic conflictual situation, a structural personality disorder, or an ongoing famil-ial pathology that hinders change in the child. He thus identifies an "at risk" situation, one that could turn into a full-fledged form of psychopathology.

There are basically two criteria by which an educational psychologist may diagnose a risk situation that requires either diagnostic assessment by specialists or psychotherapy: if, dur-ing psychopedagogical diagnostic assessment, failures emerge in specific areas of development (emotional, social, cognitive) or if, *a posteriori*, there is evidence that medical and psychope-dagogical treatment carried out at school and/or at home has failed.

In keeping with the orientation of Anna Freud and Winni-cott, it appears that the educational psychologist talks of risk when environmental and educational procedures are not suffi-ciently effective in modifying the defenses organized around either neurotic anxieties and conflicts or more profound person-ality disorders rooted in environmental deficiencies that have arrested or disharmonized the maturational process during an early phase of growth. (The risk situation, according to the educational psychologist, seems similar in some cases to a pre-psychotic or pre-structural clinical situation [as defined by psychodynamically oriented authors of the French school] which involves both the risk of evolution towards psychosis and the possibility of an evolution towards normality, bearing in mind the child's polymorphism and transformation as far as the environment is concerned.)

CLINICAL CASES

The families of children who have been advised to undergo a diagnostic assessment prior to possible psychotherapy contact the Center directly for the first consultation. At the same time or at a later date, the educational therapist separately presents a written or verbal psychopedagogical profile of the child, drawn up with either the class teacher or the remedial teacher. The diagnosis and subsequent choice of treatment carried out at the Center are described in detail in Chapter 1.

In the first two cases that follow, of two small patients and their mothers referred by the school, the educational psychologist requested a clinical diagnostic assessment for the children; at the same time, having identified a risk situation on the basis of criteria cited earlier, he helped to motivate the family towards psychotherapy. A description of the therapy undertaken in both cases is preceded by a brief psychopedagogical diagnostic profile and by an account of the treatment carried out in the scholastic environment. In the third case, there was no contact with the school, as the family came to the Center on their own initiative. In this instance, parallel treatment in separate settings was chosen for the child and the parental couple.

Ettore and His Mother

Upon the advice of the school's educational psychologist, mother and son come together to the first appointment. They are received by me and the female psychologist who will undertake the child's psychotherapy.

Ettore is in second grade but makes very little progress and has pronounced behavioral and relational difficulties. He had already been reported as a difficult child by his first grade teacher because "he keeps to himself and doesn't want to play with his schoolmates; he refuses to study, behaves in a regressive manner, and uses infantile language." An individualized and graduated teaching program had little effect on his learning abilities and socialization. This program was sustained by psychopedagogical treatment of the child that aimed at easing his feelings of mistrust and insecurity and containing his crisis of impotent rage, and also by support and information given to the mother.

Apart from the child's psychic problems, the educational therapist pointed out the manifest presence of disturbed aspects in the mother and the mother–child relationship. The 44-year-old mother works as a nurse in an orthopedic center. The fourth child in a family of five, all the rest boys, she lost her father when she was 17. After a two-year engagement to a man who "didn't want to get married," she was 33 when she met her future husband who was eight years her junior. After a one-year engagement, she married him and went to live in her mother's house. Two children were born from the marriage—Ettore, 7, and Daria, 5. Despite continuous quarrels about her husband's appalling behavior (illegal jobs, an extramarital affair with an older woman initiated while she was pregnant with Ettore) she had always refused to separate and consent to divorce; it was the husband who finally left her when she was expecting the baby girl. Ettore was 2 years old at the time.

The mother describes her son as restless, rebellious, moody, and violent like his father. Ettore's behavior during this first interview doesn't correspond to her description. Instead, hidden under a large hat and behind a thick pair of glasses, he seems to be a very shy and insecure boy. Important elements in the child's history are the following: delivery took place fifteen days postterm after a pregnancy frequently disturbed by quarrels with the husband; the baby was breast-fed for a few months and weaned at the right time; there was a slight delay in sphincter control. Ettore only went to nursery school for a few days, as the mother had problems getting him there. It was his attendance at school that first brought out or set off the psychic discomfort of the child who, according to the mother, up to that point had had no problems in the family.

At the end of the diagnostic assessment, we propose two separate and parallel therapies to the mother and child, once a week. I supervised the two therapists. Below are revisions of their reports.

Ettore's Therapy

At the beginning of the therapy and for many weeks Ettore refuses to come into the room; he hesitates when he has to take off his coat, and never takes off his hat. By so doing he communicates his total dependency on his mother, his fear of separation, his attempt to protect himself and keep himself together. At each session he controls his separation anxiety by making his mother give him food and gifts before he comes in, and by stealing small objects from the therapist before leaving. Phobic traits (fear of the devil, ghosts, monsters) as well as omnipotent defenses against persecutory anxieties (Ufo, Robot, and Big Jim, who kill all the animals) emerge during his games, which are conducted in a very confused and unstructured manner.

During his first year of therapy, Ettore repeatedly enacts his aggressiveness as if wanting to expel all the bad things he has inside ("He uses thousands of dirty words, calls me a thief, foul bitch, bad witch, because I try to stop him. . . . He breaks the plane that he often steals at the end of the session and brings back to the next session, he dirties everything, tables, walls, me . . . destroys everything he can lay his hands on in the room") and refuses all interpretations ("He puts his hands over his ears, kicks and tries to shut me up by putting tape over my mouth"). The only thing the therapist can do is contain the child, implicitly reassuring him by her constant presence over a period of time that she does not reject him and resists his attacks.

As transference slowly takes place, the child is more receptive to interpretations and gradually becomes aware of his impulses, emotions, and feelings: curiosity, possessiveness, and jealousy are sometimes discharged even before they emerge consciously, and are sometimes felt and verbalized ("You're mad, I've discovered your secret, you're married and have two children. . . . All the rooms are mine, no one else can come in or I'll kill you"). The therapist feels that an important turning point is reached when she is able to firmly resist the child's attempts to command and tyrannize her, simultaneously interpreting his desire for a father who can contain him when he feels so angry and destructive towards his mother.

During the second year of therapy, Ettore, instead of enacting his fragmentation anxiety, begins to show his need to be kept together (he lets someone help him do his puzzles), and instead of actively creating confusion, asks to be helped to *put his thoughts in order* (to arrange his figurines in order). At the same time, he begins to express friendly feelings towards the therapist and increasingly to communicate with her through symbolic activities (playing and drawing.) At the end of the second year, terrifying unconscious fantasies about the phallic and castrating mother of the preoedipal phase and about the combined parent figure begin to emerge. The elaboration of his oral and anal aggressiveness and his oedipal jealousy facilitates transition to the phallic phase. Simultaneously, he makes reparation attempts towards the object and himself, for instance when he tears up sheets of paper so that he can have the pleasure of sticking them back together again, or when he builds model cars or motor-cycles by himself.

The Mother's Therapy

From the very first sessions the woman reveals an immature, infantile personality dependent on her own mother, with whom she lives, and on her brothers (two older and one younger, all married with children), who seem to have taken the place of her father after he died. She remembers that when she was a child and her parents frequently quarreled over money, she always stood up for her mother, even though she was "very attached" to her father. During adolescence she felt very controlled and restricted by her mother and brothers in her relationships with her peers. She considered her marriage (at 34) to a man whose behavior was questionable an act of rebellion and a way to escape from her brothers' control. She did, however, want to go on living near her mother, to be protected by her husband as by a father, and to devote herself to her children—perhaps in an attempt to re-create an accepting and reassuring environment to cope with the anxiety arising from threats of persecutory external and internal objects. The husband fell short of her expectations and, after a period of repeated quarrels and mis-understandings, left home.

In the first phase of therapy, the woman spends the whole hour repeatedly attacking Ettore, comparing him to his father due to his unstable and rebellious nature. She feels she is a victim of her son and is unable to avoid being tyrannized by him. In fact, the woman has a contradictory attitude towards both of her children: she overprotects them but rejects them when she senses that they are her infantile parts, from which she cannot separate and with which she cannot negotiate. She sees them as a burden that becomes unbearable when she realizes that they are different from her, that they have their own needs and rhythms of growth. She also shows herself to be ambivalent and intolerant towards her job as a nurse. In order to appear better than her colleagues she lets the nuns who run the hospital where she works exploit her to the point of then having feelings of rejection and guilt towards her patients.

During a second therapy phase, she still discusses Ettore's problems during the session, but begins to use part of her hour to talk about her relationship with her brothers and their wives. She refuses her brothers' advice to find a new house since she is being evicted (a clear invitation to change), and asks them for money. She regards their refusal to help her financially as an attack; similarly, she feels that her daughter's teacher is persecuting her by asking her to take more interest in her daughter's studies. Burdened by challenges she is unready to meet, given the fragility of her self, she leaves her job and regresses into the family environment, devoting herself to her children and asking for protection from her brothers. She tries at the same time to patch things up with her husband and even involves his family but, once again, he leaves her and she fiercely accuses him in front of their relatives and children. Disappointed, she seems to be looking for a job again but in fact refuses a number of concrete proposals and spends the summer with her brothers, sisters-in-law, and the children, from whom she is unable to part.

When she starts therapy again in September she goes back to work and meets a man—an old friend of the family who is leaving his wife—and begins a relationship after informing her own relatives and her ex-husband's mother. She is afraid of a

new failure and struggles against her dependency and possessiveness in an attempt to let this relationship evolve positively.
Her search for familial consensus and protection coincides with
a phase of healthy dependency on the therapist, who is no longer
used just as an object into which she can pour her complaints,
but is conceived as a person who, through empathy and the
ability to understand her, helps her grow. With her therapist she
is now able to freely and shamelessly face the sexual problems
she has with her new partner.

Comments

It is interesting to note *the parallelism in the evolution of the two
therapies*. The mother begins "to think" and to recognize small
changes in herself at the end of the second year of therapy, the
same period in which Ettore stops enacting his internal world
(which coincides, to a certain extent, with his mother's) and
begins to express his needs, to elaborate his own aggressiveness,
and to assume a reparative attitude towards his therapist. The
improvements in the two therapies reciprocally influence each
other.

Often one gets the impression that it is the child who urges
the mother to keep a link with therapy, for instance, when he
refuses to come into the room if his grandmother brings him
and his mother misses the session. This can be considered as a
difficulty in separating from the mother but also as a desire to
change together and improve their relationship through the
therapeutic experience each has with his/her own therapist.
Parallel to his therapeutic experience, Ettore, while dealing with
his jealousy of his mother's companion, establishes a relationship with him that helps to improve his own relationship with
his mother (by identifying with the positive traits of the paternal
figure).

Maria Antonietta and Her Mother

At the suggestion of the school's educational psychologist, Maria Antonietta comes to the first appointment accompanied by her mother.

This is the child's psychopedagogical profile, presented in a separate session: since the age of 6 she has displayed psychic discomfort and a series of learning difficulties. She still shows reduced socialization skills (she doesn't withdraw, but only visually and emotionally participates in class activities) and learning difficulties, especially in the logico-critical area relating to the organization of verbal and written thought as well as mental relation-association processes. Psychopedagogical treatment of the affective and cognitive areas has led to a lesser degree of isolation in the class group, but severe problems remain in the area of cognitive learning.

Work on the mother is limited to making her aware of her daughter's emotional difficulties, to the point of getting her to accept psychotherapy at the C.G.C. During the first interview with me and the female therapist who is to carry out the child's psychotherapy, the mother gives us a list of detailed medical data to which the child silently listens, attentively and with interest. The story, completed later by information and details which the mother communicates during her therapy, is included to give an idea of the cultural influence of her native environment and the traumas she underwent.

Elvira, 44 years old, is a stout woman with brown hair who comes from a family of farmers. The second to last of six children, three boys and three girls, she had a difficult childhood marked by the war and the dramatic and sudden loss of her father when she was 8 ("the same age as M.A.") after an ingestion of fava beans (acute hemolytic anemia can be caused by the ingestion or inhalation of the pollen of the bean). Her 80-

year-old mother lives in her native town with two bachelor sons, her first and third children (the latter suffers from "nervous breakdowns"); the second son and Elvira's younger sister are married and live in London. Approximately three years ago Elvira lost her elder sister, hemiparetic after a cerebral ictus due to kidney insufficiency uncontrolled because of an obstinate refusal to accept dialysis.

Elvira lived at home with her parents until she was 28; she worked the land ("I drove the oxen together with my mother and brothers"), while her sisters ("all spoilt, especially the youngest who was only 5 when our father died") did needlework in the house because "the townfolk thought it was dishonorable for women to work outside the home." At the age of 24 she began a relationship with a boy from her native town who emigrated to England. After four years she abruptly broke it off when, during a visit to her brothers in London, she found out that her fiancé was having a relationship with another woman. Offended and very embarrassed, she preferred to move in with her cousins in Rome and begin work as a maid in a family rather than go back to her hometown.

When she was 32 she met her present husband who was slightly younger and worked on a construction site; her husband's family, originally from the country, was made up of a mother and two children, a boy and a girl, born during the mother's second marriage. Before the wedding a year later, her husband had a serious accident at work followed after five months by an operation for a brain hemorrhage and consequent lengthy hospitalization. Once married, the couple took a position as doormen and the woman, while continuing to work, also assisted her husband through his long convalescence.

Elvira and her husband have two children. Rodolfo, now 12 years old, was born one month premature and was very late in learning to speak. He is described as being very closed, introverted, inhibited, and a slow learner, easily subject to colds and bronchitis.

Maria Antonietta, now 8, was born fifteen days premature, "as a companion for Rodolfo and to please my mother-in-law." Kept under observation for three days because she was underweight ("she was so small and had such minute fingers"), the girl was bottle-fed since she was allergic to her mother's milk. At ten months she began weaning with no problems (she refused the bottle and preferred a spoon), but she was late teething and talking, and still uses childish language.

At the end of the diagnostic assessment we propose separate psychotherapy for mother and daughter, in the hope that any possible future change will impact positively on the rest of the family. The following accounts are revisions of the reports written by their therapists, whom I followed as supervisor.

The Mother's Therapy

The mother has a dignified and well-groomed appearance and an expression that is at the same time both hard and diffident but not lined by pain; traumas and hardships seem to have toughened but not overwhelmed her. During the early sessions she hardly ever smiles and almost never abandons her defensive attitude. She begins the first hour by saying: "We are healthy people, in body and spirit, and go to church every Sunday." She also says: "I solve my problems by myself and if it weren't for Maria Antonietta I wouldn't be here. She is a lazy child; at school they tell me she doesn't study, but she's very intelligent, a spirited and lively girl who's happy with everyone."

During the first phase of therapy she often arrives late (professing urgent engagements), and thwarts every attempt to put her into contact with her emotions and needs. The issues she does bring up are of a practical nature: the fact that her husband might be fired from his company, payment of the mortgage on an occupied house bought four years earlier, the repeated eviction deferments, the expenses for the children "who never go without," while she allows herself only the bare necessities. The sessions revolve entirely around her symptoms, her children's problems and the problems she has with them, the recriminations and demands she makes of her relatives, to whom her husband doesn't stand up strongly enough. The mother talks to the therapist as if she were reporting symptoms to a doctor or asking advice from a lawyer. (During the first three months of therapy she suffers from migraine and vertigo on weekends, and accordingly undergoes constant medical check-ups. She also reports two episodes of drug intoxication, which indicate how she personally tried to control the excitement and rage caused by her frustration and abandonment.)

Gradually, in transference, the therapist becomes a reliable and constant mother to whom she can bring her dependency needs (formerly shifted onto medicines) without feeling humiliated or rejected. Feeling sustained and understood allows her, furthermore, to retrace the painful events of her childhood and adolescence and to relive them with intense emotional participation. During the session immediately following the Easter holidays she sadly reports her fear of/desire for pregnancy; she later states that Rodolfo was born prematurely on New Year's Eve, while Maria Antonietta was born "to please my mother-in-law" on the same day as her birthday. One can suppose that giving birth to a girl on her mother-in-law's birthday fulfilled the fantasy that she herself was reborn to a richer and more available mother than the one she remembered, who was always worried and weighed down by pregnancies, financial problems, and mourning.

The work carried out during the first six months, especially the elaboration of separation, loss, and death, leads to a substantial improvement in the woman's way of relating to her children (who are given more freedom), her husband (who is less discredited and more involved in the therapy), and her relatives (in particular, her mother-in-law.) Gradually, she clings less to practical problems as expressions of extreme dependency and fragility of the self, and develops a capacity for introspection, reflection, and imagination.

Maria Antonietta's Therapy

Maria Antonietta has big dark eyes and long, well-combed black hair. The first two pictures she draws show a beautiful blond girl—her idealized self-image. Her clothes are neat and tidy and this points to her mother's interest in her daughter's appearance.

When playing, she builds a beautiful house with a laid table and a garden full of flowers, inhabited by a mother, grandmother, and eldest daughter (herself), and a maid (the therapist) who takes care of the shopping and lunch. She is often brought to the first sessions a little late and uses most of her time to prepare the toys; she puts all the flowers and trees upright, as if to consolidate, under the therapist's reassuring eyes, skills acquired through imitative processes. The fantasy of being grown-up, which characterizes the early playing sessions, seems to come from a desire to please her mother by assuming her given role; it also constitutes a defense mechanism against feeling small and needy compared to the therapist.

Subsequently, during a number of sessions, she uses only the building blocks, starting on a table far away from the therapist and gradually moving to another nearer to her. She tries to build towers that fall down, perhaps a first attempt to communicate her insecurity and fragility to the therapist. It now appears that her more infantile and needy part can be let out. She picks up a baby doll, nurses it, caresses it, but then makes it pick up large building blocks ("she has to do things by herself to learn; otherwise how will she cope when she's older?"). In a particularly significant session she seems to express all the affection and trust she has for her therapist by making her a flower-doll.

The now visible pregnancy of the therapist seems to threaten the atmosphere of confidence and collaboration that has been established. Maria Antonietta again goes to play alone on the table furthest away. She expresses intense jealousy as well as her fear of being abandoned and confused with other children (she repeatedly makes sure that the therapist keeps all her drawings). She communicates an intense fusional desire in her games, which is also apparent when she moves from a frontal to a lateral position next to the therapist whom she embraces tightly as if wishing to get inside her. The intense possessiveness towards the mother-therapist gives rise to persecutory anxieties and need for reassurance. She gives the therapist two drawings of herself: one is of a very thin, emaciated little girl, and the another of an elegant blond girl who speaks many languages and is wearing lots of jewelry.

Comments

For Maria Antonietta's mother a space was created in which she could share the responsibilities of her family with the therapist as well as recognize herself as a daughter–patient in a non-collusive and non-enacted relationship. She gradually begins to think about herself and her relationships, to work through unresolved conflicts and unelaborated losses. The fact that she had two premature births over the holiday season seems to represent a desire to anticipate childbirth on the one hand, and, on the other, to give birth to idealized images of herself as "overinvested external objects" (Khan 1974). Her intense narcissistic cathexis as a daughter can be interpreted either as a defense against depression or as a way to receive affection and approval from her mother-in-law. Therefore, it is possible that there was no "maternal capacity" (Winnicott 1958) and "parental capacity" (Giannakoulas 1983) to create the potential space in which a mother can affectively and imaginatively meet the child's gestures, a space in which the child's true self can emerge together with his ability for playing, imagining, and dreaming (in other words, using symbols).

Maria Antonietta can bring into the therapeutic space her most authentic needs and relive, in transference, the seriously traumatic and distorted early experiences of her relationship with her mother in a new way. Finally, the therapist's pregnancy enables the child to participate in the psychological change that takes place in the pregnant therapist and leads to primary maternal concern. She can also participate, through identification with the baby, in the environment the therapist creates for her own child.

Fabio and His Parents

The choice of treatment is dictated by the way in which they come to the first appointment—all three together driven by an urgent request for containment of death anxieties.

The first interview, carried out by me and the male psychologist who is to become the child's therapist, is centered on the description of the boy's congenital cardiac malformation and his medical examinations, including two brief hospitalization periods necessary to exclude the possibility of an operation. The here-and-now state of anxiety and alarm is justified neither by the child's medical condition since he is presently in good health nor by the reported reason for which a psychological examination was requested—a dysgraphia which interferes with his scholastic education.

The boy, a second child with a 9-year-old sister, was born at the end of a pregnancy marked by abortion threats during the third month, and bottle-fed due to the mother's hypogalactia. His cardiopathy was diagnosed when he was only 1 month old. His weaning period, psychomotor development, language acquisition, and sphincter control were all regular. Unlike his sister he didn't want a pacifier, has always had problems sleeping, and still cries at night if left alone. He began going to nursery school without any apparent reaction to separation from the family. His parents recently transferred him from a private to a public school, believing the latter to be more qualified to offer assistance to the child. Fabio is described as a sensitive boy, very attached to his father who often takes him out so that he can let off steam: "outside his own home, in the neighborhood, he's everyone's friend, the mascot of all the boys and his father's friends."

Following a long engagement, Fabio's parents married ten years ago, four months after the death of his mother's father. His mother remembers her sick father as totally dependent on his wife; she describes herself as having become independent from her mother at an early age. Between the ages of 20 and 24, before she married, the mother worked as a typist. Both of Fabio's father's parents are alive. He is employed at a newspaper and works irregular hours (night shifts), which means he's not at home at weekends.

Simultaneous treatment is proposed in separate settings and with different therapists—two for the couple and one for the child. The psychodynamic psychotherapy of the parental couple, carried out according to the theoretical concepts formulated by Dicks (1967) and Teruel (1966), permits us to: offer containment and transformation for the death anxieties and destructive aspects of the parents imploding in the child; favor the reappropriation of split aspects of the parent's personalities projected into the child, progressively transforming the couple's unconscious collusion and prompting the individuation process of which collusion is the negation; favor, via transference, the gradual working through of mourning and conflicts with their respective parents. A psychologist and I conducted the therapy of the parental couple. I supervised Fabio's therapist, and revised the material he made available.

Couples Therapy

The well-dressed, amiable young parents are what you would call a nice couple. This picture contrasts with the child, who is a plain boy with a thick pair of glasses, long arms, large hands, and a thoughtful expression far too serious for a boy of his age.

The couple's collusive fantasy, which emerges from the very beginning, influences their reciprocal (unconscious) choice and is responsible for the rigid boundary of the *dyadic membrane*: they collude by creating between themselves (that is within the couple) an idealized parent–child relationship in which the wife is the dependent and needy child and the husband the omnipotent parent who controls and protects the couple from anything, external or internal, that is perceived as a threat to its equilibrium. The birth of their daughter does not seem to have affected this balance. In other words, it doesn't seem to have exceeded the threshold of the *dyadic boundary*. The daughter, now 12, is described as a calm and sensible girl ("more grown-up than her mother"), and is felt to be a communal mother who stirs up jealousy in the excluded third party. The male child—with his illness, needs, and gender—introduced into the family the element of a strongly conflictualized mother–child relationship (which had been avoided up to that point in order to maintain the collusion), and made both parents face their own highly ambivalent relationships with their respective fathers.

Very quickly the mother reveals her feelings of inadequacy in the maternal role as well as her refusal and guilt towards such a difficult child. The father, instead of supporting the mother, tends to take the child away from her, partly to relieve her and partly, on another level, to avoid his own claustrophobic anxieties (in fact, he often speaks of a sense of constriction which makes him escape from home.) The couple reproduces in transference the atmosphere that maintains the collusion: they are both "good children who cannot disappoint their parents." Their aggressiveness and protests are indirectly expressed through the child, and are more pronounced before the therapeutic breaks or when the demands of the environment cause crises of adaptation and lack of confidence. When they comment with a mixture of relief, triumph, fear, and worry that "today, our son is breaking everything in the other room," it is easy to sense that, in the other room, the excited and aggressive aspect of the mother–child relationship is being enacted.

In time, the parents differentiate between themselves and with the therapists. The mother reveals herself to be more dependent and trusting, and she uses the therapist better in the sense that she feels emotions and verbalizes and discharges them; she accepts the interpretations that sustain her desire for growth, but rejects those centered on her regressive desires. The father is more introverted and tends to rationalize, deny, and make things banal; in fact, he seems to have a fragile and fragmented self and appears to be more resistant to change. While his wife meets change with fear but also hope, he considers it catastrophic even if it seems favorable.

The transference evolved from holding to dependency. Even if there is strong resistance to the interpretative work aimed at recuperating infantile parts of the self projected into the child,.

and elaborating the unconscious aspects of the couple's relationship and transference relationship, the work does gradually favor identification with the therapists: the mother prepares the child's schoolbag, sews his pockets ("one, I couldn't manage two"), makes him be punctual, and tries to frustrate his greed; the father, identifying with the male therapist, learns to support his wife instead of taking her place, and his tendency to escape outdoors decreases, signifying reduction in the persecutory aspect of his internal world.

After approximately a year and a half of therapy, the husband is offered a more challenging job which requires his presence in the office, together with other people, as well as his acceptance of a role of dependency on his boss and more time with his wife, since he will now be free on weekends. After discussing the pros and cons for many sessions, both decide not to pass up this new moment of growth. But in fact, the father's new job disrupts the family and the change creates anxieties that are enacted in therapy; for instance, since the husband can't take time off from work, the mother has to get herself organized to bring the child to sessions and comes late. Once this difficult moment passes, the couples therapy begins again on a regular basis, after a two-month hiatus which negatively affected the child.

A new crisis occurs when the daughter leaves the family for the first time, creating abandonment anxieties in the parents, especially in the father. The interpretation of the separation anxieties, more pronounced at every therapeutic break, permits the gradual elaboration of the separation and individuation of the parents from each other and from the children. Before the summer holidays the mother, pleasantly surprised, tells us that the child, who never wanted a pacifier, has asked for a teddy bear.

Fabio's Therapy

From the very start, Fabio brings to therapy all his destructiveness, fragmentation, confusion, and greed; he breaks everything and wreaks havoc. His stories tell of lonely children who are afraid of everything and bad children who kill. During the first sessions, he appears to be frightened by the damage he causes as if the therapy room were the mirror of what is happening inside him: the attacked objects persecute him, the ink spots disgust him, the newspapers suffocate him, so that he is forced to climb up onto the window to escape. His father is presently the object of his aggressiveness ("I want to kill Daddy"). By often playing a game in which he blacks out the room, he dramatizes the anxieties and fears that overcome him at night in bed (the wolf who eats him, Dracula, death); the darkness during the session conjures up these terrifying images but at the same time creates an atmosphere of intimacy that allows him to communicate them to the therapist.

With the Christmas holidays approaching, the themes of death and abandonment present at the start of therapy re-emerge: again Fabio talks of lonely children betrayed by their mother, or of a dead mother. At the same time, he undergoes medical exams (blood sampling and dental treatment) that give rise to fears of being emptied of vital parts and to an intense production of complicated, terrifying stories, full of skeletons, monsters, and blood-sucking vampire-snakes. For Fabio, the therapy room is a place where he can discharge anxieties, impulses, and fears; only many months later—after having repeatedly verified that the therapist has survived, is waiting for him, and is not vindictive—does he become affectionate and trustful, to the point of falling asleep during therapy.

During a session that takes place immediately after the Easter holidays, he screams and shouts because he was left alone: he swears, takes it out on everyone, claims his mother let him die and his father is shit, and sees the therapist as Dracula. In the same session, through dramatization, he communicates his desperation at not being able to possess the object and his terror of being imprisoned within the object and within himself; for another entire session he tries to remove one cube stuck inside another, and during the next he shuts himself in the cupboard, which becomes his tomb. The fact that he is able to express all his hate for his parents who "made him ill" and recognize the violence of his intrusive fantasies as well as his desire to protect the therapist, marks the start of a collaborative and reparative attitude towards the therapist. In fact, he spontaneously helps him to tidy up the room with increasing frequency.

In September of the third year of treatment, a relatively quiet period, Fabio makes considerable progress in therapy, in the family, and at school. He tries to separate, by doing a series of gym exercises to become stronger, which he repeats during a number of sessions; he begins to show interest in his "doctor" (he draws a picture of him near a tank full of fish) and to distinguish between good and bad objects (fairies and monsters). Each time holidays or events occur outside the immediate family (his grandmother's illness, the eviction notice), they represent a threat to the integrity of his self and produce temporary regressions, but they do not affect his confidence or hinder the evolution of the therapeutic process. The child begins to contain himself on his own, for instance, when he asks for a diary "to write down my thoughts and understand the passing of time." He is less confused, speaks more clearly and, at the same time, at school there is an improvement of his dysgraphia. Although he shows intense jealousy towards other children (putting up signs to mark his territory), some of them become pleasant playmates whom "the colt doesn't want to leave to go home to mother." Finally, ambivalence towards the therapist is expressed in the frequent mood changes that occur during sessions.

Comments

Of the numerous considerations which come to mind when comparing the evolution of parallel therapies, I will illustrate here, for the sake of brevity, only one aspect that I consider interesting, namely, *the response of the parents to environmental pressure involving an internal change and its influence on the child*, who represents their most fragile and needy part and, at times, coincides with the damaged and persecutory internal object of both.

During therapeutic breaks, or when the father found a new job, or the eviction notice was served, we noticed that:

- The mother regressed and sometimes had somatic reactions; the fantasies of emptying and dirtying the object and, consequently, the persecutory and abandonment anxieties decreased.
- The father resorted to omnipotent and autistic type defenses; in transference, the therapists were envied and denigrated, and his claustrophobic anxieties become more pronounced.
- The grandparents have been, in fact, involved in a supporting role and this provokes fear of exploitation in the mother and a feeling of anger and humiliation in the father.

The child's therapist, if he wanted to understand and interpret correctly, had to keep, so to speak, two sets of books: the evolution of his relationship with the child (as described in the child's therapy), and the intrusion of the parents' internal world into the child's and the defenses the child activated in order not to feel overwhelmed and threatened in his integrity. As his trust gradually increased, the child expressed himself better: for example, he was able to communicate by playing when the claustrophobic anxiety related to his fantasy of intruding into the object (he climbed *into* the cupboard), or when his feeling of being stuck was because he felt either crushed by the projective identifications of his parents or identified with an expelled fecal persecutory object (he slid *under* the cupboard).—cf. Pallier 1984. The therapeutic relationship evolves, in the sense that instead of acting out to reduce tension or to communicate by playing or dramatizing, Fabio begins to express himself verbally and to associate freely: "grandmother is ill, daddy is going to play football, mother's tired, and I'm tired and hungry."

CONCLUSION

Having established the importance of the school in fostering the global maturational process of the child, I will briefly outline the importance of obligatory schooling as a social structure complementary to the family that offers the child the possibility of having "other" experiences and the parents the opportunity to delegate some of their educational and formative functions.

Scholastic education and socialization are successful when the emotional and mental growth ("from dependency to independency," as defined by Winnicott) reach a level that permits detachment from parental objects and investment in other objects, or when the child, even if affected by personality or behavioral disorders in the family, succeeds in taking to school a functioning or healthy area of his personality while the family remains the receptacle for, or may even foster, his sick part. In this case, the school, rather than the family, can become an *alternative* and more suitable environment to encourage the communication and development of symbolic activities because it represents the "different from self."

The difficulties encountered when the child first goes to school arise if "the other than self" constitutes a threat for the fragile and fragmented self of the child, or if the demand for scholastic performance represents a burden for those children whose difficulties and symptoms were compensated for, tolerated, or even maintained by the family (in support of homeostasis in the family system). In these situations, the school acts, so to speak, as a *detector*, becoming an important preventive tool in the psychic disorders of children and adolescents.

My experience teaches me that in many cases the school workers are equipped to assess and carry out the psychopedagogical treatment necessary to help the child overcome his or her emotional difficulties. In only a minority of cases were the environmental procedures implemented by school workers, either in school or in the family, insufficient to restore affective and cognitive development in the child, such that referral to a specialist center was considered appropriate.

There are certain advantages to conducting psychotherapy in a center for psychic disorders in children and adolescents located outside the school boundaries. Treatment, even if initiated by the school, requires the active involvement of the family, whose motivation has to be strong enough to overcome the disincentives of having to make contact with the center and having to respect a waiting list. The center's separateness avoids confusion in the patient and greatly reduces the internecine conflicts that arise (between the school staff and the psychologist and educational psychologist who work in schools) when the psychotherapy is carried out by the school's psychologist.

The element of motivation and the establishment of a

therapeutic couple and a setting (one hour per week for an indefinite period) initiate a process that constitutes a therapeutic experience, since it brings about changes in the patient's ego and self, or, in other words, a psychoanalytical psychotherapy, thanks to the creation and evolution of transference (cf. Petrella 1982). The parallel treatment of the mother or parents is based in particular on the theoretical assumption that the child's pathology is closely related to the quality of his/her early experience with the mother (cf. Giannotti on the pathology of the self in children, 1981) and/or to a pathology of the parental couple unable to offer a holding environment capable of fostering affective and cognitive development in the child.

As I attempted to establish (and generalize) certain criteria defining the analytical psychotherapy carried out at the C.G.C., I realized that the most common theoretical reference points applicable to the territorial situation in which we worked were those inspired by the formulations of Klein, Bion, and Winnicott. From the comparison and discussion of cases followed for a minimum period of two years, it has emerged that our therapeutic process evolves according to the following pattern:

1) There is an improvement in the threshold of tolerance to frustration and a reduction in the tendency to acting. From the very beginning, by having to wait for their turn and not being able to substitute one therapist for another, many people learn to tolerate the frustrations of waiting and respect the setting.

2) There is a change in the person's capacities for feeling, understanding, and thinking. During the first phase, the patients tend to discharge onto the therapist all their feelings and emotions, in other words, to rid themselves of the emotional complications involved in human relationships; only later do they become aware of the experi-

ence of emotional contact with themselves and with others, and reduce their tendency to satisfy their need for love, understanding, and mental growth exclusively through economic well-being (Bion 1962).

3) There is a reduction of the confusion that often results from an inability to tolerate frustration and the tendency to complicate situations in order to phobically avoid those tension zones that an immature and imperfect ego is unable to bear.

4) Self-sufficiency gives way to the possibility of benefiting from psychotherapy. It is the "capacity to use the object" (Winnicott 1968) that "favors transition from a stage of ruthlessness to one of concern" (Winnicott 1954) or to a depressive position, as defined by M. Klein (1935, 1940). Only after having learned to use the therapist can Ettore and Fabio pass on to the reparation phase.

5) A potential space is created in which patient and therapist can play together and in which the patient can develop his/her imagination, fantasy, and ability to use symbols. Originally, this was the potential space between mother and child in which the child could experience his own omnipotence before realizing its illusory aspects.

6) The possibility of two therapeutic settings—one each for the mother or parents and child—permits the creation of two spaces, at once facilitating the separation-individuation process and underlining the aspect of collaboration.

While the assistance the school gives a child is part of the school environment, at the Center parents and children come together to improve their relationship and grow. The cases presented in the first two chapters highlight the school's pivotal role in identifying psychopathological risk situations and encouraging motivation in the families in addition to the importance of our being able to make psychoanalytically oriented psychotherapy publically available.

A number of questions now spring from the critical review of the cases followed over a seven-year period. Compared with spontaneous motivation in the family, is the motivation promoted by the school an unfavorable prognostic element as far as the effectiveness and (relative) rapidity of the treatment is concerned? Is a family's motivation towards the child's psychotherapy linked to social class or to the type and gravity of the child's/parents' pathology? Would the patients sent to us by the school have ever initiated psychotherapy in a public health service or private practice on their own and if so, when?

The fact that more cases were sent by the school than presented on their own leads me to put forward the following general considerations:

- Compared to families who came spontaneously to the Center, those families motivated by school workers needed a longer period of time to shift their dependency from the school to the therapeutic relationship. For instance, during the first phase they tended to interrupt therapy during school holidays, as they considered the C.G.C. an appendage of the school. This took place even in those cases in which there was no specific defense against dependency, such as that of considering the therapist a teacher and the session a lesson.
- Generally speaking, the families who came spontaneously to the Center presented more serious pathologies than those sent by the school.
- Some families referred by the school who belonged to a low social, economic, and cultural class would not have sought psychotherapy for their children's psychic discomfort if it had not been presented by the teacher or

educational psychologist in an accessible and appropriate language form—specifically, as a sort of assistance that (since it does not "concretely" satisfy dependency needs) neither fosters dependency nor underlines the shame and humiliation of being in need, and requires active participation.

The last two points above implicitly stress the school's preventive function in the psychic pathology of the child, in terms of both coming first and exposing a wider range of the population to the possibility of psychotherapy. Of course, psychotherapy, unlike other second level interventions in which the local services play a similar preventive role, is based on free choice and a desire for mental and emotional growth; therefore it cannot be prescribed.

3

PARENTAL INVOLVEMENT IN DIAGNOSIS AND THERAPY

When dealing with adults, the diagnostic interview that aims at establishing objective criteria indicating the need for psycho-analytical psychotherapy takes into account the patient's psychopathology and his motivation for psychotherapy, and the psychotherapist's experience and theoretical inclinations. A child, however, can undergo and benefit from psychotherapy whatever his pathology and quite apart from motivation, which is initially difficult to assess.

If the therapist is able to establish the therapeutic alliance with the parents and maintain it throughout therapy, the child will, sooner or later, develop his own personal therapeutic alliance.[1] I have only rarely seen a child refuse diagnostic inter-

---

1. D. Meltzer writes, in *The Psychoanalytic Process* (1967):

the analysis of children should reveal the analytical process in its purest form. Not only does the child come to analysis innocent of cultural misapprehension as to the nature of the process, but he takes to it unselfconsciously and without conscious motivation. . . . the analytical views, psychotherapy, or analysis if it is presented correctly and if the parents are convinced of its importance or significance. I let the child participate in the first interview with the accompanying parent or parents to lessen his fear of the "different from self" and also to give him the opportunity *to communicate with me in the presence of his parents or with his parents in my presence*, precisely because he feels I am different from both himself and his parents. From the start, the child seems to understand the role of the psychotherapist and communicates his problem through verbal expressions; he externalizes intrapsychic conflicts in interactions with the parents or in other behaviors for which consultation has been requested.

Following the first joint session, there are a number of individual diagnostic interviews with the child and parents. Often, what appears to be a real disposition of the parents to cure the child very quickly turns out to be merely their own need to be reassured and to understand what is happening *to the child* rather than *to their relationship with him*. This occurs even as early on as the diagnostic interviews. In such a case, the consultation ends with the parents requesting advice and the therapist hoping that some comment or testing interpretation, addressed to the child or one or other of the parents, might produce an insight and start a self-therapeutic process.

This kind of situation, even in instances where the child

---

process takes him into its realm unawares. . . . it is not reasonable to speak of their being uncooperative either until a clear alliance has been developed in the adult part of their personality. . . . [p. xv]

In the treatment of psychotic children, however, since one starts with a non-integrated ego condition, one cannot speak of a therapeutic alliance in the classical sense as an object relation that favors the mobilization of relatively independent resources of the patient's ego (Zetzel and Meissner 1973). Clearly, one may speak of therapeutic alliance when a sufficiently structured cohesive self is established (Lanza 1986).

needs psychotherapy, is less traumatic for the child and less frustrating for the therapist than one in which the parents, initially available, later threaten the child's therapy with actions and complaints that may lead to its interruption, perhaps just at the very moment they perceive a change. At that point, often neither the therapist's experience nor his determination is sufficient to re-establish a therapeutic alliance.[2]

The idea of involving parents in therapy came from the need to guarantee a stable therapeutic setting for the child by removing the environmental pressures that acted and continue to act as a traumatic factor on the child, interfering with his potential growth as restored and freed during psychotherapy. Later on, the importance of the idea was confirmed by the fact that, frequently, either the request for consultation and therapy for the child or the lack of collaboration during the child's therapy could be interpreted as *a defensive attitude of the parents against a personal* (from the parents themselves) *unrecognized or denied request for help*. Only in certain circumstances were the attacks on the child's therapy considered a negative therapeutic reaction of the parent towards an improvement in the child.

In the C.G.C., I immediately tried to create a physical and mental space for the parents: the parent's room. The fact that a number of psychotherapists worked in the service allowed me to offer not only support but proper psychotherapy of one of the parents or parental couple, which could begin at the same time and take place either parallel with the child's therapy or at a later date.

Questionnaires were never handed out to the parents because we did not want them to consider our work an institu-

---

2. The therapist's experience includes his ability to accept transference and analyze countertransference, with regard to both the child and to his parents.

tional routine, and we did not want to create an inquisitive context promoting guilt or non-guilt or to fuel passive expectations or pathological dependency attitudes and behavior. Particular attention was paid to the parent's motivation towards *involvement* in treatment. A setting was established for the child and for the parent with the assurance that no other patients would be received at that time and day.

The mother rather than the father spontaneously involved herself with the treatment, willingly using her space and therapist; she was also relieved and pleased that the child worked in a different but adjoining space, with another therapist who was in contact with her own. This made me reflect on the fact that if this parallel setting was accepted as a methodological proposal, it was also correctly perceived as an invitation for all involved to assume their own responsibilities while at the same time remaining in a context of relationship and an atmosphere of collaboration. The message the family seemed to receive was: everyone has his own space (i.e., aspires to personal individuation) while trying to live together as well as possible. In other words, the fact that the therapists worked in separate spaces in the same institution and were in touch with one another encouraged the gradual growth of the embryonic identity and differentiation of each family member in psychotherapy as well as the integration of the family group and development of a feeling of belonging through mirroring with the group of therapists.[3]

---

3. A. Correale (1991) identifies in the institutional therapist group a very specific group state which, in itself, constitutes the equivalent of the chaotic and fragmentary demand in the patient's family group. I found that if the team of therapists is made up of the therapists of the child, mother (or father) and parental couple, and if the confusion and fragmentation of the family group are received and contained by the group of

When I reflected on this experience in the National Health Service, I realized that, instead of adapting the analytical approach to institutional requirements, I had tried to transpose an analytical setting into a public environment, exploiting the advantage the latter offered me in that it is a service which hosts a number of workers. The constant effort to distinguish the approach and objectives of the psychotherapies from other health and welfare services carried out in the district, as well as the time limits and the need for organization and coordination with the other services, did, however, present remarkable disadvantages when compared to private practice. Often the patient who turns to the psychologist or psychiatrist working in public health services tends to identify him with the service itself and, in turn, to associate the psychotherapy service with the wider context of public health and welfare services. The fact that treatment is free permits intervention in situations that would never have reached private practice but excludes the economic element as an important motivational factor. Why, then, not apply this parallel therapy technique in private practice since it proved to be so successful, especially in those cases that presented a severe psychopathology that would have been difficult or even impossible to tackle by simply conducting individual therapy of the child without promoting a family change?

FROM PUBLIC TO PRIVATE

The above considerations encouraged me to assemble independently a group of trainee psychotherapists in child and adult

---

therapists and transformed through the elaboration of the relationships between the therapists, then the family will be able to introject more mature and disciplined group function modes.

psychotherapy, so as to be able to offer parallel analytical psychotherapy to children and parents in my private practice. Among the benefits of having a team of psychotherapists when working with children, adolescents, and severely affected patients are the capacity to treat severe pathologies more successfully, since these require the therapy of more than one family member and an in-depth study of the collusions that sustain and nurture the patient's disturbance, and the capability to study the family and intervene therapeutically without compromising traditional psychoanalytic concepts and techniques (dyadic relationship, setting, exploration of profound dynamics).

I transposed the methodology with which I had already experimented in the public service into a private practice, with modifications. Once the diagnostic phase was completed, at the time of the contract, I proposed therapy in keeping with an evaluation of such criteria as the type of pathology, the readiness or refusal of the parents to accept parallel therapy, and the level of preparation and theoretical inclination of the therapists. The proposals called for either analysis of the child three or four times a week plus regular interviews with the parents conducted by the child's therapist, or parallel psychotherapy of the child and the mother (or father) with two different therapists two or three times a week—as well as an additional space for the parental couple, to take shape as: (a) regular interviews by the child's therapist with the parents (generally before the holidays) in cases where the objective was simply to maintain the therapeutic alliance or explore couple dynamics, or as (b) couples therapy conducted by a third therapist in cases where the parents wanted to face the problems in the marriage as well as the problems of the child. In situations involving preadolescents or adolescents, the parents were referred for support interviews to a therapist other than their child's. Couples therapy or the parallel therapy of either one of the parents was suggested only in instances where the pathology (of a parent or of the parental couple or of the family) permitted the therapist to foresee even during the diagnostic or contractual phase that the parents would be otherwise unable to protect the child's space and that the child would be unable to accept a relationship with a person outside the family.

Particular care is taken, in public services and, to a great degree, in private practice, to formulate a therapeutic proposal that corresponds to real motivation on the part of the parents and therefore guarantees the therapeutic alliance. The proposal that establishes on whom and how frequently to act must consider such risks of collusive behavior on the part of the person formulating the proposal as: passive compliance excluding the father, ratified by cultural stereotypes based erroneously on the negation of the father's emotional need; complicity with the parents' tendency to turn the child into a scapegoat and with the child's omnipotent tendency to assume this role; and complicity with parental delegation of any parental role to the child's therapist.

THE PARENTS' RESPONSE
TO THE THERAPEUTIC PROPOSAL

Now that a number of years have passed, I am able to illustrate some results of my therapeutic undertakings, with collaborators, in both public and private settings.

- In most cases, parents preferred to be involved instead of letting the child go through personal analysis independently. In only a few cases did the parents allow the child to undergo analysis and limit their involvement to just a few interviews with his analyst: this was the choice of those who presented genuine motivation for the child's analysis. They were mainly parents with neurotic or more serious pathologies that did not, however, interfere with the parents' capacity to establish and maintain a therapeutic alliance with regard to the child's therapy.

- In general, the mother appeared to be more available to undergo parallel therapy, while the father—identifying with his culturally codified role—preferred to sustain the economic burden of the therapy and leave the introspective work to the wife. The father was more absent in the public sector than in private practice.

- Being able to carry out sessions simultaneously was correctly interpreted as a way of taking into consideration the family's needs, avoiding the discomfort of numerous and sometimes long journeys.

- In cases of psychosis and infantile autism, two simultaneous therapies in parallel settings were preferred, in addition to a third setting for the parental couple, who regularly had interviews with the child's therapist. The fact that the therapies of mother and child go on at the same time and in the same place is important in order to avoid an initial drastic separation between mother and child; such a separation could be traumatic in cases of fusional symbiosis and consequently result in a strengthening of the pathological symbiosis. Giannotti and De Astis (1989) propose a common initial mother and child setting for the same reasons.

- In most cases of adolescent therapy, the parents acknowledged the significance and usefulness of entrusting the child to the therapist and putting up with exclusion, or of limiting contact with the child's therapist to the initial phase of therapy. Otherwise, they accepted referral to a second therapist for regular or occasional interviews, as long as the two therapists were in contact with one another.

The *connection* between the two therapists becomes a *transitional area* between the child's therapist and the parent's, which corresponds to the need for transitionality between parents and children in the separation–individuation phase of the adolescent. In the case of psychotic adolescents, the family was involved through the creation of more than one setting in an attempt to break the collusions that maintain the fusion and confusion between the various members of the family.

4

SUPERVISION OF
PARALLEL THERAPY

My supervision of psychotherapists conducting parallel therapies in separate settings for several family members provided me with a vast body of clinical material concerning the therapy of the child, the mother (or father), and the parental couple— material that had to be reconsidered and interpreted in the service of better understanding and transmission.

In proposing an observation model that would embrace the therapy conducted in each setting, the way the therapists coordinated their work, and the supervisory function, I have tried to break down the investigation into component areas.

- Observing the evolution of the internal object relationship according to the "natural history of the analytic process" as defined by Kleinian theory—splitting, splitting and idealization, projective identification, unconscious phantasies, internal objects, part and whole objects, and so on (Klein 1932, 1946, Meltzer 1967)—and of modifications of narcissistic personality structure, toward either acquiring a coherent basic structure or transforming a pathological narcissistic structure into one that is less pathological (Kohut 1971).

In other words, both the narcissistic and drive dimensions of personality are considered alongside the development of the corresponding types of transference in the corresponding settings. According to Green (1983) all clinical material can be understood from the narcissistic vertex and the object vertex even in situations that are not particularly narcissistic.

- Considering how a relationship arises between patient and therapist through the creation of a transitional area.

Winnicott added to Klein's concept of internal object relationships the concept of an intermediate area of experience between what is purely internal and what is purely external, and argued that it is in this area that one enters into relationship with the object. And Bollas, in a lecture at the University of Rome's Istituto di Neuropsichiatria Infantile in 1987, remarked that "it is easier for the analyst to think about patients only in terms of internal objects, while it is harder to find in the analyst a part dedicated to observing and working through the intermediate area, that is, to observing the atmosphere that has been created with the patient, the interchange, and himself at play with the patient." Bollas went on to say that this "second aspect of the analyst's work is equally important since, in a certain sense, one of the analyst's tasks is to foster the transition from internal object relations to relations between two persons."

- Identifying in the child the effects of past traumas and the impingements of mother and environment in the early stages of the construction of the self: to use Green's (1983) terms, discovering in the child a discourse that alienates

him, a discourse from outside him that overlays his own
discourse.

In metaphorical terms this means evaluating the mag-
nitude of the damage caused by earthquake (strong trauma
or impingement), by slow infiltration of water or air
pollution (cumulative trauma), by work stoppage (withdrawal of libido cathexis) in a city under construction—
the child's emerging self.

• Identifying crossed projective identification that creates
  confusion between mother and child, distorts communication, and opposes the process of separation and indi-
  vidualization.

  When child and mother (or father) undergo therapy at
  the same time, the two therapists can observe their interactive style—modes of relating that are intrusive, adhesive,
  or autistic—both before the patients enter their respective
  therapy rooms and after their sessions, as they leave. The
  analytic process conducted in each setting fosters the
  transition from narcissistic to introjective modes of identification.[1]

• Listening in the two settings to the experiences of mother
  and child regarding the child's efforts to separate from
  mother and hers to separate from the child, while at the
  same time working through anxieties and defenses about
  separation from the object in the transference.

• In the marital setting, observing changes in the couple and

---

1. Ferro (1987) argues that while the natural direction is from patient
to analyst, there may be projective identification between analyst and
patient even in normal situations.

I share Bollas's opinion (1989) that projective identification is a
two-way process in the mother–child couple and also in the analytic dyad;
that is, the analyst acts on the patient by way of projective identification,
influencing his internal world.

shifts in the transference and relationship of the parents towards the child's therapist at the time when the child is changing, thanks to therapy or to his own growth drive.[2]

All the elements that have thus far emerged were collected and elaborated separately by each therapist.

Having mother and child sessions *at the same hour* has proved to be a useful technical parameter, because meaningful communications can be collected by the two therapists in the waiting room before and after sessions, the only time they meet both patients together.

The extemporaneous exchange of ideas by the two therapists (mother's and child's) after the sessions fosters additional observation and thought, as to the degree to which mother's emotional states, linked to traumatic events or contingent frustrations or the emergence of conflict, influence the emotional states and behavior of the child and vice versa, and also as to how both mother and child react to external events involving the whole family (like a move or a death).

Methodical comparison of the two sessions might even make it possible to assess whether there are stable correlations between the mother's different mental states—manic, depressed, autistically withdrawn—and the state of the child's self. In one clinical situation I can think of, when the mother brings in a cold split-off aspect of the self, the child acts "crazy" in his therapy room; when the mother spews complaints and protests the whole hour, the child brings a fragmented self to his therapy and asks to be held together.

---

2. Marital therapy is conducted after the model of Dicks (1967) and Teruel (1966) as developed in the Marital Unit of the Tavistock Clinic, London.

Integrating the clinical material from all three settings in the course of supervision makes it possible to focus on features of *collusion* between mother and child, father and child, and parental couple and child that impede the individuation and evolution of the therapeutic process in the respective settings.

At discussion sessions, colleagues have pointed out that the position of sole supervisor of two or three therapies—child's, mother's, parental couple's—raises some inconveniences that might invalidate the very work my proposed model intends to develop, or even challenge the therapeutic value of parallel therapy. They have contended that supervision conducted separately by a single supervisor over therapists conducting parallel therapies might foster the transmigration of material from one therapy to the other without the supervisor being aware of it, and such transmigration might seem to confirm clinical hypotheses *a priori* and prematurely.[3]

I believe, however, that although single supervision may not guarantee rigor in the research or heighten the quality of therapy, it makes possible—once the setting is established after the assessment phase (concerning what family members should be involved and how often) is complete—the emergence of a *dynamic field* in which the supervisor becomes a *participating observer* of the therapeutic project in its entirety.[4] The resulting field is broader than the bi-personal one that is set up in the analytic situation, and it is complicated by the intense affective dynamics activated among all the members of the therapeutic

---

3. I am grateful to Maria Assunta Di Renzo for raising this objection and stimulating further theoretical thought and reflection.

4. The idea and the field model applied in the analytic situation have been studied by Baranger and Baranger (1961–1962), Corrao (1986), Correale (1986), Bezoari and Ferro (1991), and Neri (1993).

team, each with his own role and functions. From the vertex of the single supervisor it is possible to focus on one or another of the analytic relationships without losing an integrated and unitary vision of the clinical material, of the complex transference and countertransference phenomena, and the relational dynamics activated not just between patients and therapists but also between therapists and supervisor.

I hope that the assessment of clinical material from different settings, the careful attention to how the therapists receive the supervisor's intervention, and the supervisor's responsibility for what continues to happen in the field, including the supervisor's countertransference (Ferro 1992) may elevate the demands on attention and emotion that constitute the challenge of managing the complex therapeutic set-up I have described to the dignity of a clinical and methodological contribution. It seems to me that the technique of parallel therapy opens up new prospects for deepening knowledge of the psychic disorders of children and parents and their unconscious interaction. Its implementation should make possible the extension of psychoanalysis even to those serious pathologies of child and parent that are considered to be at the limits of analyzability.

5

COLLUSIVE ASPECTS OF THE MOTHER–CHILD RELATIONSHIP IN NARCISSISTIC DISORDERS[1]

1. This chapter is a revised version of a paper read at the International Congress "Narcissism, Nomos, Transgression" held in Rome in 1987 and published in the Minutes.

INTRODUCTION

The previous chapter dealt with the work group I organized in order to treat, in a private setting, those childhood pathologies that require a diagnostic assessment and a psychoanalytical psychotherapy or analysis of more than one family member. The need to organize and interpret the extensive clinical material acquired through the separate supervision of each of the psychotherapists who conducted parallel therapies prompted me to establish an articulated field of research illustrating the therapy conducted in each setting, the coordination of the various psychotherapists, and the role of the supervisor. The comparison and close examination of the clinical material regarding the psychotherapies of the child, the mother, and the couple enabled me to carry out an in-depth study of the pathological collusions between mother and child. That material is the subject of this chapter.

ASPECTS OF PATHOLOGICAL COLLUSION
IN THE MOTHER–CHILD RELATIONSHIP

In Italian, *collude* has two meanings: to collude is to play together, to have a hidden alliance, and also *to have a secret complicity against another's legitimate rights.* I would like to adhere to that dictionary definition and interpret other people's rights in a psychological key—taking for granted the concept of collusion in psychoanalysis as defined by Dicks (1967),[2] Greenacre (1971),[3] Laing (1961),[4] and Meltzer (1985),[5] to mention but a few. I consider "other people's rights" to refer to each person's right to reach a feeling of physical and separate existence and recognition of self in relation to another person. I consider this the primary condition for all evolutionary, transformative, and creative movements of the individual and of the couple.

In this chapter I will examine collusion in the mother–child couple, the two family members in psychoanalytical therapy.

The collusive aspects of the child and mother against the

---

2. Dicks (1967) defines the "essential collusive process" in a more general sense, "as a reciprocal attribution of unconsciously shared feelings" (p. 68).

3. Greenacre defines *focal symbiosis* as a partial collusion between mother and child—a fairly strong reciprocal dependency limited to a circumscribed relationship; at its core is generally a pathology in the adult, but the emotional disorder is usually manifest in the child.

4. Laing (in Dicks 1967) describes collusion in married couples as a process in which "not only does the person wish to have the other as a hook on which to hang his own projections, but also tries to find in the other, or induce the other to become the very embodiment of that regressive or fantasied other whose collaboration is necessary to complete the particular identity he feels stimulated to sustain" (pp. 127–128).

5. Meltzer uses the term collusion when referring to the *folie à deux,* which he defines as a relationship whose content is incidental to the strength of the bond: the two persons are bound by a double system of projective identification on two different levels, genital and pregenital.

father and other family members are explored in the setting of the parental couple, and inferred in the therapeutic relationships of the child and the mother through the use of transference and countertransference. It appears to me that the collusion between mother and child in neurotic situations (particularly pronounced immediately prior to analytical separations), may be interpreted according to the "playing together" definition. The mother projects needy aspects of her self onto the child in a way congruent with the states of the child's self, and satisfies them by taking care of the child. She also projects onto the child instinctual aspects that she may either control or frustrate in the child or deal with him in a play area, while bringing her own dependency needs to her husband. The child accepts his assigned role, exploiting the secondary advantages of regression. The father contains his wife's dependency needs, and recovers his own dependency needs towards her by identifying with the child. The Oedipus conflicts of the father and mother towards their respective parents are dealt with in the child–mother–father triangle, according to the level of elaboration (pregenital and genital) of the Oedipus conflict reached in therapy by the mother and child.

To examine the pathological relationship between mother and child in those cases in which the mother presents narcissistic personality structure and the child produces symptoms that reveal either his own suffering or that of the mother–child couple, I will refer to the three defensive narcissistic structures described by Sassanelli (1982):

- *the ideal self* or idealizing narcissistic structure;
- *the antilibidinal self* or antilibidinal narcissistic structure;
- *the parasitic grandiose self* or symbiotic-parasitic narcissistic structure.

Three categories of selfobject correspond to these configurations:

- *the ideal selfobject,*
- *the repulsive selfobject,*
- *the depository selfobject.*

Sassanelli's structural approach to narcissism provides a theoretical reference point that confirms the significance of some of the questions that repeatedly come up in my own clinical studies. In which area of the personality of the mother with a narcissistic pathology does the disturbed child fit? Why does the disturbed child simultaneously threaten and maintain the mother's narcissistic equilibrium? Is the psychic disorder of the child already inscribed in the mother's unconscious in the sense that the child is assigned an unconscious signification even before birth? If the function of narcissism is rooted in two complementary sequences—to permit the globalizing representation of oneself and to ensure self-preservation—how can the real child be accepted without threatening this function? Can the mere presence of the child as an other than self, as a real child, represent the destabilizing factor effecting a pathological defensive organization of the mother?

According to Sassanelli the psychic world is populated not only by mature representations of the self and the objects, but also by more archaic images that belong to various evolutionary stages and levels of integration, starting with an undifferentiated primary matrix (Mahler 1968) or psychophysiological primary self (Jacobson, 1964). "A fundamental task of narcissistic structures is to control these immature, deviant, or altered psychic formations, which can damage or seriously threaten the stability, continuity, and cohesion of the whole personality" (Sassanelli 1987, p. 506).

Using Sassanelli's language and passing from the narcissistic mother to the narcissistic mother–child relationship, one can say that *the mother with a narcissistic personality structure includes the child, the selfobject, in her defensive narcissistic organization, or else that she projects or displaces onto him those deviant (damaged, highly needy, or falsely powerful) images that the narcissistic structure tries to control.* If the child is unable to find in another member of the family, namely his father, an object that recognizes his right to exist and satisfies his dependency needs, then the child colludes with the mother according to patterns I will describe shortly.

The classification that follows, based on my clinical experience, indicates where the child is placed in the personality of the mother with an idealizing type narcissistic structure, the mother with an antilibidinal narcissistic structure, and the mother with a symbiotic-parasitic structure, as well as how the child colludes with the mother in the case of each of these personality types.

The Idealizing Narcissistic Structure

If the narcissistic structure of the mother's personality is ruled by an ideal self, the child could be the *ideal selfobject* with which the ego of the mother makes a pact to deny the destructive part of her personality (the internal saboteur or antilibidinal self); alternatively, the child may coincide with an internal object to be repaired omnipotently by the omnipotent dimension of the mother's personality (ideal self). The mother unrecognizes or frustrates the needy libidinal self of the child, just as she unrecognizes or frustrates her own. It has seemed to me that, in many cases, the mother recognizes and accepts only the needy component of the child's infantile self (the small, defenseless child), not the impulse component. The child colludes either by accepting the role of ideal selfobject unable to disappoint the mother's specific expectations or by containing the projection of the mother's damaged objects, which sometimes places him in dangerous situations that stimulate an omnipotently reparative activity in the mother.

The Antilibidinal Narcissistic Structure

For the mother with a personality in which an antilibidinal type defensive narcissism is dominant, the child becomes a *repulsive selfobject* with which the mother's ego allies to defend herself from the more archaic, deviant, and damaged parts of her internal world; alternatively, the child corresponds to damaged internal objects to be destroyed. The needy libidinal self of the child is rejected. If the child who represents the mother's repulsive selfobject does not accept the projection of the anti-libidinal aspect, he is deprived of every physical, mental, and emotional contact. In both these defensive configurations there is a minimum amount of independence and individuation of the object, but the object must have that role and that function; in other words, *the child is cathected by the mother only if he is placed in the area of her specific fantasies.*

The Grandiose Narcissistic Structure

For the mother with parasitic *grandiose self*, the child's role is to immobilize perverse and psychotic elements of the mother's personality (that correspond to Bleger's [1964] ambiguous nucleus or Bion's bizarre objects): he becomes a depository selfobject or buffer. "The relationship of the depository with the grandiose self is totally mirror-like in the original sense of the term, in

-other words, fusional, and their link is a parasitic one that establishes a symbiotic identity" (Sassanelli 1987, p. 509).

CLINICAL ILLUSTRATION:
MOTHER AND CHILD IN SEPARATE
AND PARALLEL PSYCHOTHERAPY

Alessio, a mute autistic child, began analysis with me at the age of 5. Four years later, his mother, affected by narcissistic personality disorders with borderline functioning, started psychotherapy with a female psychotherapist in the same practice and with the same time schedule. This case illustrates the difficulties in managing the relationship with the parents until the mother was motivated towards personal therapy, and in treating primitive mental states at preverbal and presymbolic levels such as those of a mute autistic child.

I met Alessio, now a good-looking young boy of 13, for the first time eight years ago. His parents are a handsome couple: she has brown hair and an interesting face; he is tanned, wears a mustache, seems self-confident and uninhibited. Their letter of presentation clearly states that the child has a better, more relaxed relationship with the father. And it is the father, Dante, who tells Alessio's story, while the mother, Edda, takes part only in order to correct a few points, revealing aspects of emotional instability and a marked affective inhibition.

Edda, an only child, was entrusted to a maternal aunt when she was about 2 years old and put into boarding school for several years at the age of 8, because it seemed that "at the time the parents didn't get on together." Edda's mother, described as being pleasant and remissive, was her father's second wife; her father, who died of a cerebral ictus shortly after meeting his grandson, Alessio, is depicted as having been possessive and jealous. Edda, after graduating from high school, pitted herself against her father and met her future husband, Dante, abroad. Until he married Edda, Dante lived with his father following the marriages of his brother and sisters and his parents' separation, which took place when Dante was 25.

Edda and Dante lived together for four years and separated just before the birth of their child. The pregnancy was normal despite the mother's solitude and the birth full-term (anesthetic during expulsion, artificial milk feeding). Alessio was left with the grandparents for a short period when he was a few months old. He began to walk when he was 18 months old and was urinary incontinent until the age of 4. Up to a few months before consultation Alessio had some special habits: "he only touched or put in his mouth things that had previously been touched or tasted by his mother, and he also bit continually." The child is presently going to nursery school and appears sufficiently integrated with the other children. He does not talk (he pronounces only certain repeated syllables to name his mother and father) and is very "fussy." He has tantrums if he doesn't get his own way and "cuddles up tenderly to his mother before falling asleep."

Alessio's first session takes place in the presence of the parents. He is a pretty, blond 5-year-old whose eyes are at times fixed and dazed, at times shifty, like his mother's; he is hindered in his movements by an unsteady gait that I cannot place in any known neurological syndrome.

It seems to me that Alessio is regarded by his frightened and guilt-ridden parents as someone who controls everyone and everything, like an old grandfather who cannot be contradicted. Based on the medical data and direct observation of the child with his parents, I now realize that what was considered a better relationship with his father is, in fact, an imitation-compliance type behavior superimposed on an avoidance attitude towards his mother, a mother who could not hold the child in her postnatal womb (Tustin 1972–1961).[6] They were a mother and child who, in all likelihood, could not use each other to recuperate the narcissistic wound caused by the birth in both the child and the mother (Giannotti and De Artis 1989).

Dante, who now has a new family, and Edda, who has worked since her own mother moved in with her and Alessio, decide to let their son start psychotherapy three times a week. A brief narrative of the first phase of that and of the development of my relationship with the mother and the parents, up to the point four years later when therapy was interrupted for approximately a year and a half, follows.

The First Phase of Alessio's Therapy

From the very first sessions, through his gestures, noises, and bizarre destructive behavior, Alessio immediately made me feel immersed in his confused, chaotic, and psychotic world. By endlessly repeating an activity that consisted of a continuous transfer of toys from one basket to another with one or two variations on the same theme, Alessio communicated the nucleus of his autistic pathology—that is, his attempt to avoid the experience of being separated from his mother by maintaining the illusion of a spatial-temporal continuum, by preserving the distorted illusion of a fusion with the mother–sensation-object (Tustin 1981), his omnipotent fantasy of keeping his and his

---

6. In a conference held by Dr. Tustin at the Institute of Infantile Neuropsychiatry in Rome (1987), Dr. Fè d'Ostiani pointed out that the mother of a psychotic child does not hold the child "in the uterus of her mind" but in an autistic nucleus of her personality that contains intense and sometimes terrifying fantasies and experiences. The child feels threatened by these malignant narcissistic fantasies contained in the mother's black hole as if they were a real danger, and reacts with withdrawal and freezing.

mother's "pieces" together, his fear that he would be left empty or that his mother would be left empty.

The concrete setting (the actual space of the therapy room and the length of the session) facilitated a change from a two-dimensional functioning of the mind, from the experience of being in an infinite space-time to the experience of being in a space-time limited in the mind of the therapist and in reality. Alessio's experience of being contained by this space rather than being emotionally reached by the interpretation of his autistic maneuvers permitted him to come into contact with his psychotic depression (Winnicott 1958).

Over a considerable period of time, during every session, Alessio would flood the bathroom and throw things on the floor and out of the window. At the end of the session, he would put his whole hand in his mouth. By doing this, he tried to control "the terrors of falling, of dissolving, of spilling" (Tustin 1990, p. 59) of feeling "the black hole with the nasty prick" (p. 301). These terrors were connected to a state of indifferentiation and to an adhesive quality of the relationship with the object.

At a later stage of therapy, he would reach the capacity to deal in a play area (discovering of the door, the cuckoo game) with the anxieties connected to the awareness of the separate existence of the object and to separate himself from me, knowing that he could think of me and be confident that he would see me again. This implies that the differentiation of the self from the object has been achieved and that a psychic space has been created in the subject. This space contains the representation of the object and the internalization of the link with it.

Gradually he came out of his sensorial world. If I asked him to stop, or even if I merely looked at him disapprovingly, he stopped stimulating himself anally by rotating his buttocks on the basket and orally by noisily sucking his soft palate. He also demonstrated that he had acquired his own tools to regulate the flow of violent sensations and excitement by closing the faucet by himself when the water level rose above a certain height. He began to express emotions and communicate through mimicry and gestures. The mimicry and the stereotyped gestures, as well as his bizarre behavior, were less frequent and were concentrated in the session around a sequence of actions, difficult to decode, which Alessio executed in order to pull out, by using his hands and his teeth, pieces of toys from a basket (fragments of the self confused with the non-me, partial objects, bizarre objects?). An increasing integration of his self lent support to an incipient functioning of the ego. Alessio began to do little jobs at school and listened briefly to me tell him fairy tales that I developed from pictures printed on cards that he chose from time to time.

The foregoing excerpts from treatment correspond to the standard therapy for autistic children described by Tustin. However, some of the mother's symptoms and some of the traits of her personality, as well as the persistence of a psychotic nucleus in the child (the contents of the above-mentioned basket), led me to think that a symbiotic psychosis was superimposed on the autistic disorder.[7]

During a meeting with the mother prior to summer break, Edda told me of a dream that I believed synthesized the traumatic area and revealed her incapacity to cope with it. I did not convey the interpretation of the dream to her, but instead I wrote it down together with her communications from that session, which I considered to be associations.

---

7. In symbiotic psychosis the child is trapped in the immature or psychotic elements of the maternal personality, according to Giannotti and De Astis (1989). The length and outcome of treatment are directly linked to the seriousness of the maternal (or paternal) psychotic nuclei.

The dream: "Alessio's not there. A female friend and her companion walk in front of me. Dante and I follow. I have a long, enormous thread inside me. I try to pull it out, but I hurt myself and so I leave it inside."

Associations: "The husband of a friend has had a heart attack and no longer speaks. A female friend of mine had a dream in which Alessio spoke. My father died of grief when he discovered that Alessio couldn't speak. It's really difficult for me to be careful all the time so as not to hurt Alessio, which is what Dante expects."

I analyzed the dream by breaking it down according to my knowledge of Edda at the time, and emphasizing those elements confirmed by dreams Edda subsequently referred to a future female psychotherapist.

- The dream began by declaring a loss: Alessio was not there—Alessio being either the object or the vital or developing aspects of self.
- Edda's associations connected the pain generated by the extraction of the thread with a very strong feeling of distress caused by a traumatic separation, an intense and acute pain recorded in the somatic self (friend's heart attack, father's stroke) and apparently impossible to either register mentally or express in words.
- The fact that Edda didn't move the thread in order to avoid causing the wound to bleed can be regarded as staying in the traumatic area in which her traumatized self was confused with the trauma-causing object and with her disturbed child. Edda's association linked the death of her father, due to a brain hemorrhage, with the lack of speech in the child. The child is included in the traumatic area and the mother–child collusion resides in their incapacity

to bind the pain of the "original wound" (Jungian formulation: personal communication by E. Fè d'Ostiani).

- Edda set up a link through associations between being able to talk (the friend's dream) and being able to psychically elaborate traumatic occurrences.

After hearing the dream, I felt the need to provide Edda with a space in which to bring her own needs and dreams and asked her whether she would be willing to begin psychotherapy with a female colleague in another practice. Edda declined this proposal saying that "it's my son's brain that's sick, not mine." On demand, I continued to see the mother, and, sporadically, the parental couple. While maintaining control over his wife and child—a control I considered inversely proportional to his real availability—the father refused to see me alone.

From the moment Alessio began therapy, his father, even if legally separated from the mother, continued to spend a lot of time with her and often accompanied mother and son to the sessions, so I suggested to both parents that they start a couples' therapy. They accepted, but then abandoned the therapy after just three sessions, whereupon mother, father, and child, all smiles, arrived with a present for me, a "doll with three breasts." The message, even in its pathological collusive aspect, is so clear to me that no explanation is necessary.

After a few months of therapy Edda met another man who moved in with her. She stopped working, fulfilling a regressive fantasy of finally finding someone who would take care of her completely. However, two years later, this relationship also broke down, due to Edda's excessive possessiveness and her inability to have a relationship with other people *unmediated by her son*. Only through Alessio and for Alessio did she really express her needs and aggressiveness.

The "ghost of the lost object" became Edda's guiding light for a long period of time during which she passed from one form of acting out to another, missed Alessio's sessions as well as her own, telephoned at the most unthinkable hours, and refused to pay me. Edda thus revealed to me an anal-aggressive aspect of her character consisting in rebellion and control over the object, which contrasted with the image she had previously given me of an acquiescent, respectful woman. My being patient and firm allowed her to avoid regression and escape from therapy.

I supported Edda in her decision to find a job, accepting her proposal to reduce the therapy hours for Alessio, who in the meantime had regressed and worsened, because I felt it was necessary to boost her confidence by offering an alternative to her paranoia and withdrawal. During one session he flooded the bathroom and splashed the mirror for the whole hour. At home he did "mad" things such as cutting up the carpets and laughing, and at school he dirtied himself. I believe it is important to underline that the child learned to say no when the mother began to realize that it was impossible to find someone or something to solve all her problems. (The acquisition of "no," which coincides in the object relationship with the tendency towards object constancy, introduces difference, rebellion, and desire to separate from the other.) Edda began to work and the child was sent to summer camp. It was at this point that she asked for a suspension of therapy, proposing that I see Alessio every now and then on demand until such time as she could pay off all her debt.

After a year's interruption I began therapy again with Alessio, this time adding a parallel therapy with the mother at the same time and in the same practice. Edda accepted it now because this parallel and contemporary therapy did not expose her to a traumatic separation from the child and from me, and perhaps also because she had developed some awareness of her own pathology.

Therapy of the Mother and Parallel Evolution
of the Child's Therapy

The creation of a second setting for the mother—which she immediately felt and recognized to be a private, containing, and protective space—facilitated the separation between mother and child that was already marked by the presence of "No" in the latter, and introduced new elements in the child's therapy as well. As Edda experienced her therapist's reliability and capacity for reverie, her *impingement* on Alessio—her use of him as depository of her own psychotic nucleus—diminished. *The containment of the mother's aggressiveness and destructiveness and the development of libidinal aspects in her therapeutic relationship had a structuring effect not only on the self of the mother but also on that of the son.*

A brief interruption of treatment due to the therapist's pregnancy produced a rheumatic somatization in Edda. When treatment recommenced, she worked on "re-writing the history of her relationship with her son" by empathically participating in the therapist's capacity for maternal concern. One of Edda's dreams showed her trying to retrieve Alessio's "ball" (the libidinal aspect of the mother–son interaction) from a "muddy, dirty swimming pool" (the mother's basic attitude of pessimism and lack of confidence). In turn, Alessio communicated that he accepted his mother's reparation by, for many sessions, kissing a photograph brought from home "of when he was small." At the same time, he dirtied and cleaned the mirror in the bathroom in an attempt to find a mother-mirror reflecting an image in which he could finally recognize himself as a good, accepted boy.

Alessio was happy his mother had her own therapist and developed a transference and a relationship with his mother's therapist that evolved over time. While initially he seemed to ignore her, he later took an interest in her by successively expressing attraction and repulsion, jealousy, and sadness when he left, and joy when he met her again. I could now concentrate on my relationship with Alessio and pay greater attention to the analysis of transference and countertransference, especially to the images evoked in me by Alessio's behavior, now that I no longer had to invest most of my energy in my relationship with the mother *as though the mother's therapeutic relationship represented a third entity protecting the therapeutic alliance in the child's therapy.*

Alessio could now bring me his intolerance to separation and his possessiveness and intrusiveness towards a weak and vulnerable mother not protected by a husband, his impulses to bite himself and his grandmother (for a long time Alessio kept rage out of his relationship with his mother). In other words, the representation of the child's self emerged as a nucleus responsible for impulses, actions, and feelings. Careful observation of the sequence of gestures and actions, and decoding of aggressive behavior and attacks of rage and anxieties through analysis of the countertransference helped me to direct my therapeutic strategy.

To consider or interpret splitting and fragmentation solely as the consequence of the child's sadistic oral attacks and his inability to mentalize separation from the object—and not as resulting also from the traumatic effect of the impingement produced by the projective identifications of the mother into the son, or by her inducing in him tension and behavior—might add to the child's confusion, and increase his feeling of not being understood with ensuing anger, desperation, and withdrawal. On the other hand, to attribute everything to the trauma and reaction to the trauma might prevent the child from assuming responsibility for what he does to the object, either in reality or in his imagination, and worse still, it would deprive him of the hope of being he himself the agent of change.

When Alessio pointed to himself, it was not easy to understand when he meant "this is me, I did it" or when instead, he attributed to himself an aggressive, provocative, or incongruous behavior rooted in an aggressive introject belonging to the mother's unconscious or derived from an identification with pathological aspects of the mother's personality. Alessio seemed to sense my doubts and comprehend my efforts to reach him, when, for example, he put his fingers into the electricity socket to make me understand whether the "tension" was put into him by the mother (or environment) or whether, instead, he himself acted out this destructive gesture. To signify the first, he banged the wall, to signify the second, he looked at me with a defiant air, and solicited a containing gesture.

The work with the mother, dream analysis in particular, permitted assessment of her parents' personalities and their disorders as a couple, as well as the way in which both influenced the structuring of Edda's personality and her marriage choice.

The father, a reserved man tending towards regression and withdrawal ("a bear who shut himself in his room and never did any of the little repair jobs around the house"), was unable to sustain his "depressed" wife during her pregnancy. Edda's mother's first-born son died during her pregnancy. One can suppose that Edda's mother was totally absorbed in mourning her dead son (having lost with her male child her characteristics of power, aggressiveness, and activity), and further disappointed by the birth of a baby daughter. It may be that these are the reasons Edda was entrusted to an aunt for two years and then sent to school away from home. As a teenager Edda moved to another city, without working through the separation from her parents. She chose a partner who was deeply traumatized by his mother's second marriage and who revealed himself to be unable to tolerate the birth of a child. Alessio was felt, even before his birth, to be a third party, who prevented the parents from putting an end to their arguments, and withdrawing each to their respective rooms.

Edda lived in a state of psychic immobility based on a false self and on the tangible reality that Dante was the only person who did in fact take care of her to some extent. Alessio was still trapped in the parents' pathological bond and his psychosis seemed to be related to it. The psychic paralysis was expressed in transference by constant attempts to immobilize the analytic process through the depreciation of psychoanalysis and of the transference interpretation, by the inability to associate freely and to "play," and by continually referring everything to what was seemingly concrete reality (parasitic type transference).

For the whole session Edda talked of anger with, and intolerance and rejection of her son's disturbed behavior. If, on the one hand, Edda needed to put the therapist's patience and tolerance to the test with regard to the anxieties her son caused and her wish to get rid of him, on the other, it seemed that she used her son as a defense in order to prevent the therapist from emerging as an object. Her contribution to therapy was revealed by her growing capacity to show her therapist, each time, various aspects of her self that corresponded to her defense to avoid contact with the traumatic area and the "basic lack of the object."[8]

• She could not choose the regressive "solution" previously fantasized with her second partner of a world of well-being and

---

8. E. Fè d'Ostiani (personal communication) connects the "basic lack of the object" with the emotional absence of the mother, in that, for reasons not attributable to depression alone, she cannot cathect her son. The newborn is formally cared for but otherwise rejected; his true self will register an absence of the object while the false self will maintain a pseudo-relationship with a pseudo-object. If the baby's resulting narcissistic withdrawal is complete, he may become psychotic.

prosperity in which "life is all peeled and ready." Apparently inspired by her mother, this solution corresponded to a return to the womb fantasy and was criticized by her ego as unrealistic and ridiculous. This "fetal" relationship model was reproduced in therapy—especially before analytical breaks, through a fusion type transference in which the therapist's assigned role was to function as the mother's placenta—and also in her relationship with Alessio, when Edda herself placed the son in a newborn-fetal position.

• She could not escape where perversion and promiscuity omnipotently erased the trauma and opposed reparation of the self and the object. This was the solution the husband offered when at night he smoked and drank and told her about all his problems with his new wife and suggested that the two families meet "all together passionately."

• She could not get better, as suggested by the alliance of her healthy part with therapy, since she was full of anger, rancor, and recrimination at having been rejected by two men, and loaded with her omnipotent guilt for "having destroyed her mother and killed her father by giving them a sick child." The internalization of a good experience was slowed down by paranoid projections (in one dream the two therapists appeared as "two thieving cooks") and by a basic pessimism which "drained her therapist's reserve of confidence and energy."

Edda's true self was located in her son, and the relationship between her false self and the self expelled in her son was extremely contradictory and tormented. Alessio was experienced contemporaneously as the "me" that abolished any psychic or emotional distance whatsoever between subject and object, and as the dangerous "non-me" that could destroy the survival of the false self. Alessio was, in turn, the dirty, "disgusting rat," who robbed her of all her energy and prevented her from living normally—and with whom she engaged in a sado-masochistic struggle—the incorporative greedy pig, the affectionate dog who kept her company, the controlling father, the depressed mother who invited her to regress, and her own vital self promoting growth.

Alessio was caught in a paradox of having a mother only if he accepted the role she gave him, and naturally this seriously interfered with my attempt to make him undertake a separate physical and mental existence. *Pathological identification with the mother saved him from the hostility and withdrawal he would have experienced if he had tried to differentiate himself from her.* The mother hampered the child's symbolization process insofar as she assumed the mental functions that the child split and projected onto her! Symbolization and language, with the differentiation and distance they involve, were forcefully opposed by one aspect of himself with which Alessio identified completely in his games—the "pig," who claimed supremacy over mentalization of bodily sensoriality and drives.

The analytical work on both mother and child was hindered by the *collusive aspects of the mother–child relationship* that opposed the separation-individuation process as well as verbal communication. The fact that Alessio and his mother could not sleep in their own beds revealed their inability to separate and indicated the way in which this inability was connected to the mother's relationship with her original objects. Mother and son managed to sleep in their own beds only if there were guests in the house; otherwise they were able to separate only by sleeping in each other's beds or if the mother slept in the guests' sofa-bed and Alessio in the big bed.

For Edda, apart from the true self I mentioned earlier, Alessio also represented the phallic defense that attacked dependency on the object by guaranteeing self-sufficiency and prevented her from female identification with the therapist.[9] As these were her fantasies about her son, Edda would have felt proud if Alessio had separated but, at the same time, she would have felt castrated, empty, and damaged, as illustrated clearly by one of her dreams.

Edda's capacity over a period of time to keep a bond with therapy and her vital drive, even if it was split and projected onto her son, entitled one to hope that the narcissistic gratification and self-esteem deriving from her own improvement and that of her son would compensate for the loss of the symbiotic object.

---

9. It is as if the child's body, hardened by the distorted (defensive) sensation of being fused with hard objects, was felt by the mother as a phallus ("Alessio doesn't have a stomach, he's always got taut muscles," she says) to the point of becoming at times an erect, male organ–baby, immobilized in the role of "a grandiose phallic, depository self-object" (Sassanelli 1982, p. 312).

6

PARALLEL THERAPY

It has long been known that parents' conscious and unconscious attitudes and fantasies play a specific role in the development of the child (Johnson and Szurek 1952). If account is
not taken of the connection, there can be no access to the
complete understanding of the child's pathology, nor can sym-
pathetic support for treatment be obtained from the parents.

HISTORICAL SURVEY

The means of approaching parents and involving them in the
analytic process has been an important problem throughout the
history of child psychoanalysis, starting from the first case—
Freud's analysis of a phobia in a 5-year-old (1909)—conducted
by way of the child's father.

In 1945 Anna Freud said that during the evaluation of a child
for analysis one had to diagnose and borrow the parents' ego
during a child's analysis. The analyst needs the parents' coop-

eration and must be watchful of the part they play in the resistance to resolution of the neurotic process in the child. Therefore the child analyst must deal not only with the child but with the parents as well, so that the child may be freed of infantile fixations and move in the direction of development. The analyst's efforts are often resisted by the intensity of the parents' neuroses and their effect on the child. In such cases the child does not progress *"unless the parent involved is analyzed as well"* (p. 136).

As early as 1932 Burlingham stressed the analyst's need to keep the parents favorably disposed toward the child's analysis "to prevent premature interruptions. Often the parent is unable to help the child without having been analyzed himself" (Burlingham et al. 1955, p. 165). In 1955, in cooperation with A. Goldberger and A. Lussier, Burlingham authored the first description of a simultaneous analysis of a child and a parent, conducted by two analysts who *did not communicate* with each other but brought their sessions for weekly supervision to Mrs. Burlingham in order to coordinate the material. They sought to reveal "what influences were at work and what close relations there were between the mother's unconscious fantasies and the child's attitudes and disorders." They made the interesting observation that the unconscious fantasies that originated in the mother and were then internalized by the child could be successfully handled in the child's analysis; but the destructive and seductive behavior of the mother, the acting out of her unconscious fantasies, functioned as a traumatic agent that served to constantly renew the close bond between mother and son, countering the influence of the analysis, which was working in the opposite direction.

In 1960 Ilse Hellman presented the case of 11-year-old Eric and his mother, both in analysis, as part of a research project in simultaneous mother and child analysis at the Hampstead Child

Therapy Clinic in London. And Anna Freud, in her introduction to the 1960 report of Kata Levy on the simultaneous analysis of a mother and her adolescent daughter, said that the material obtained from nine analyses of mothers and children at the Hampstead Child Therapy Clinic was of inestimable value in highlighting the points of interaction between the abnormalities of mother and child. In particular, the interaction between parent and child is fundamental for "clarifying the bases of personality and the roots of mental illness" (p. 379).

Kolansky and Moore reported the findings of simultaneous analyses of four parent–child couples in Philadelphia over a period of eight years in their 1966 paper, "Some Comments on the Simultaneous Analysis of a Father and His Adolescent Son." They cited as advantages a clearer picture of the child's developmental lines, his inhibitions, regression, and progress; greater insight into shared psychopathology and its effects; prevention in some cases of worsening pathology in the child; and the more immediate surfacing of specific tendencies as a result of the exchange of material between analysts than would be likely if the individual analyst knew only his own case. Unlike the Hampstead Child Therapy Clinic researchers, these authors *exchanged material* and overcame the difficulties of the transference and the countertransference.

Although the degree to which child analysts today work with parents depends on the analyst's theoretical stance, the nature of the child's disorder, and the inclination of the parents, there is almost unanimous agreement that, in cases of serious psychopathology, analysis of the child is not sufficient (Novick and Novick 1992). Fifteen years ago, when I began seeing parents and children in the public health service in Rome, a bibliographical survey like the foregoing had already confirmed that work with parents, including the real analysis of one parent or the other, was key to understanding the pathogenic influence of the child's environment and to removing those aspects of the parents' pathology that obstructed the therapeutic effect of the child's analysis.

I have spoken at length of my experience with parents and how my approach evolved over time, both in public and private sector work. In the course of broadening my understanding of the parents' problems and finding empathic and collaborative attitudes toward them, my interest gradually extended *from the child to the parent–child relationship and from the child's disorder to that of the parent*. So I tried to establish favorable conditions (preliminary conversation with parents, organizing a team of psychotherapists) for offering psychotherapy or analysis to parents as well. The shift in interest from the disturbed child to the disturbed parent and the extension of investigation from what happens in the inner space of mother and child to what happens in their relationship (Piovano 1987) preceded my going deeper into psychoanalytic theories that give primacy to the relational aspect of the psychoanalytic experience and the importance of the real features of the analyst and his involvement in the analytic relationship. The increasing attention paid by the analyst to the patient's observations and communications in response to his interventions seemed to be in line with my research on the mutual influence of the psychic life of parent and child.

THEORY AND TECHNIQUE OF PARALLEL THERAPY

What follows is a review of the operating model I have developed as a therapist and supervisor in the practice of parallel treatment and of its application by the psychotherapists who are part of my working group.

• The psychotherapist who conducts the assessment consultation offers the parents parallel therapy.

- A mother or father schedules therapy parallel to that of the child and with the same frequency; it may even be simultaneous (i.e., at the same hour).
- The parental couple has regular meetings with the child's therapist before scheduled breaks in the treatment. The diagnostic therapist who suggested treatment in parallel settings informs the parents that the therapists will share as much information as they believe they can without interfering with the relationship each therapist has with his own patient in his own space.
- The therapists have the same supervisor, who collates the material from the different settings. In some cases the therapists conduct parallel therapy without supervision, except at the early stages of the experience, and they meet for discussion among themselves instead. (In the early stages of my own experience I conducted one therapy, usually of the parental couple, while at the same time supervising the therapists who conducted the parallel therapies. Now I refrain from being part of the therapeutic team when I act as a supervisor, although I do supervise therapists working with family members I have seen in assessment consultation.)[1]

The technique of parallel psychotherapy offers advantages both cognitive (expansion of the field of observation of psychoanalysis) and therapeutic (expansion of the field of application of psychoanalysis), which compensate for the intense organiza-

---

1. Experience shows that in the advanced stages of parallel therapy, the parental couple has sometimes returned to give me information about the progress of the child's therapy or to consider marital problems emerging in the course of it in conversations with the child's therapist. This signals motivation for marital therapy, and emerges when the child's problem is on the way to being solved but the parallel therapy of one parent has not modified the pathology of the couple.

tional and emotional efforts required to develop it. They comprise essentially the possibility of

- Enhancing the understanding of each case by way of going deeper into the contribution of external reality to psychic reality (not only real events but, more important, the real objects that constitute the child's current relational context[2]), and going deeper into the ways in which real interpersonal events are worked through in psychic reality and in which phantasy makes use of real traumatic events (Del Soldato and Ferrara Mori 1985, Gediman 1989).
- Assessing the pathogenic role of the parents' personality in the genesis of the child's disorder.
- Exploring the unconscious aspects of parent–child interaction with particular attention to collusion, which prevents the parent from establishing the distance requisite to implementing adequate parental functions and reinforces the child's sense of omnipotence and false self, preventing him from taking the role of child.
- Observing how the family is transformed through modification of interpersonal relations and the process of destructuring of the "field of family pathology" (Neri 1993), which starts from the intrapsychic changes of the family members who undergo therapy in parallel settings. Change in intrapsychic aspects is reflected in family relations and family structure.

––––––––––

2. Rosenfeld (1987) recommends careful examination of the family interrelationships and attention to the role that the analyst plays in transference. "I now try as much as possible to assess the patient's relationship to her or his past and *present* environment and so to lessen the possibility of confusing the healthy and sick part of the patient" (p. 270).

SIMULTANEOUS PARALLEL THERAPY OF CHILD AND PARENT AND THERAPEUTIC CONVERSATIONS BETWEEN THE CHILD'S THERAPIST AND THE PARENTAL COUPLE

Parallel therapy conducted at the same hour and in the same venue proved to be the preferred setting in cases of child psychosis and autism. In the here and now of the session and throughout the duration of the therapy, it facilitated exploration of the reciprocal influence of mother and child, with particular reference to the traumatic impact of the mother's mental and emotional life on the child and vice versa.[3] Conceptually the focus shifts from the effects on the child of an early failure of the environment to the *current* situation of *mutual traumatic action*. The trauma is no longer regarded according to a logic of linear causality, whereby parents and environment are deemed responsible for the child's pathology (Nicolò 1989). Instead consideration is given to the possibility that the mental functioning, defensive structure, fantasy-making, and changes of the mother have a traumatic effect on the child, that the child's archaic mental functioning may reveal or activate depressive nuclei and psychotic scars in the mother. (This latter possibility is experienced by the mother as a threat of destructuring her psychic apparatus.)

Simultaneous parallel psychotherapy also offered an opportunity to probe the collusive aspects of the mother–child relationship, which impede the analytic process in both settings.[4] A

---

3. Bonaminio, Carratelli, and Giannotti (1990) suggest exploration of the areas in which the experience of the real relationship and fantasies about the relationship overlap.

4. Sandler (1990) cites internal resistance linked to collusion with the mother that prevents the child from collaborating with the analyst and

dynamic process is set in motion in the double setting, which includes the sensations, emotions, affection, fantasy, and thoughts of the four people involved in the analytic situation (child, child's therapist, mother, and mother's therapist). That process is articulated at various stages.

First Stage

Mother and child arrive together.

The therapists receive them together in the waiting room and can catch aspects of their relationship that have emerged since the last session and will be communicated in this one. I refer, for example, to intrapsychic conflicts acted out in the mother–child relationship (mother and child arguing when they arrive), or behaviors connected with early traumatic experiences (original scars, denied mourning) that mother and child mirror back and forth or compulsively repeat because they have never been worked through and thus are unassimilable and "unthinkable" (Tagliacozzo 1982).

An example may clarify this point. A mother arrived very anxious because her son had run off just before the start of the session. This episode was interpreted as a dramatization in a shared space—the waiting room, in the presence of the two therapists—of the trauma of a brusque rupture of the fusion with the primary object. Further, this same trauma may be relived, narrated, and historicized at different tempos and in different ways within the two therapeutic relationships.

---

the treatment. "It is not sufficient explanation," she says, "to attribute the child's difficulty entirely to his conflictual transference with the analyst" (p. 25).

We shall see in the next chapter that on the occasion of treatment breaks, the child enters fairly early into contact in his therapeutic relationship with the psychotic anxiety connected with separation and otherness and the loss of the object. The mother tends to try to manage these anxieties within the relationship with the child by acting out on the child and using him defensively, until the initiation of the therapeutic process and the emergence of transference phenomena modify her deeper mental structure. The mother, by way of projective identification, may make the child feel imprisoned and immobilized— anxieties connected with *her* conception of the link of analytic dependency—or she may expel into him her true self, the source of her anxiety and rejection, or traumatic areas not worked through in which the child's self, her own injured self, and the object responsible for the trauma are confused.

Each couple works in its own room.

In each setting it is possible to integrate the pathology of deficit with that of conflict. That is to say, it is possible to determine whether the clinical material is rooted in *deficit pathology* (failure of the environment, failures in development) or in *conflict pathology*, by assessing the quality of the transference (defensive transference, defensive resistance, conflict-transference, deficit-transference); by analyzing fantasies arising from the sadism that determines the paranoid distortion of early parental images (Kernberg 1984); by analyzing the countertransference, facilitating re-creation of early traumatic states (Bollas 1987a); by assessing the nature of the anxiety (anxiety about the fragmentation of the self, or anxiety about the loss of the object, the object's love, or castration) and the response of the patient, to orient the therapeutic strategy.

In the adult, structural deficits arising from early traumas have been organized over time into conflict structures, giving rise to character patterns so complex that, while derived from deficit, they are no longer distinguishable from those derived from conflict.

"Even where the component of deficit dominates the pathological make-up and accordingly an affirmative quality [based on empathic understanding of the trauma] has to be built into most of interventions, this will not be sufficient. Analytic interventions will be needed to unveil resistances and to explore the fantasies in terms of which the patient has reinterpreted reality" (Killingmo 1989, pp. 73–74), and also to address the distorted components of the subsequent reworking and reinterpretation of early traumatic experience in which unconscious phantasy and introjects play an important role.

In the child, early traumatic relations are easier to determine and reconstruct. That is to say, *the access to the original area of the trauma is more direct*.[5] The trauma, however, is not simply registered as a cathectic hole to be filled or as a wound to be healed. The primary aggressiveness and secondary hatred (anger, vindictiveness, disappointment) that grow out of deprivation and lack of emotional cathexis lead to alteration in the child's emotional needs which are thus ambivalently structured and give rise to extremely persecutory internal and external object relations. Unless the child's aggressive resistance is re-

---

5. Scholars who consider trauma from an interpersonal perspective root early traumatic relations in environmental failures that have undermined the basis for the construction of the self: traumatic failure of the reverie function (Bion 1962); failure of the mother as protective shield (Khan 1974); failure by objects that have not met the child's developmental needs (Tolpin 1971); his needs for symbiotic fusion (Mahler 1968, Mahler et al. 1975); his need for basic self-assertion (Kohut 1978); absence of structuring unconscious fantasies and/or presence of unassimilable unconscious fantasies in the parents (Bonaminio et al. 1989).

peatedly identified and interpreted, excessive rancor toward the mother prevents the child from accepting reparation from the analyst (who is assimilated as the mother), or from the mother herself as she gradually changes, thanks to her own therapy.

Mother and child take leave of their respective therapists and depart together.

It is surprising to watch the mother in the waiting room "learn" from the child not to fear contact with the trauma and anxiety triggered by parting, and at the same time "learn" from the therapist not to hide from the child at parting.[6] Mother and child identify with the therapists and gradually trust the link and the possibility of maintaining the link. Often in the case of psychotic children, the mothers' stories are constellations of mourning, conflicts, and traumas that have not been worked through. In the psyche of these mothers the basic wound and subsequent traumatic experiences have been recorded as blind spots. They may show themselves clinically in the way the mothers avoid getting in touch with their own and the child's separation anxieties, which avoidance reinforces the child's efforts to keep the mother always present by plugging the hole with autistic objects or other people who are not distinguished from the mother.[7]

---

6. The concept of saying good-bye and then meeting again presupposes a long process of learning in childhood. Learning what it means to say "good-bye" and to meet again is a conquest that requires time and entails some neurotic pain in even the healthiest individuals (Rosenfeld 1992).

7. Due to the specular quality of the experience of mother and child (Tustin 1990), a mother who has experienced the birth of a child as an amputation, as the loss of a protective part of her own body, will not be able to help the child when he realizes that the nipple, from which he

The therapists talk after every session.

A spontaneous exchange of ideas between the mother's and the child's therapist after each session helps to assess how and to what degree emotional reality, mental processes, and the state of self of the mother and child influence each other. Methodical comparison of sessions helps to assess whether there are stable correlations between the mother's mental and affective states and child's states of self and behavior. If, for instance, the mother is victim of a depressive crisis, the child may react by flight into manic behavior or autistic withdrawal, or he may attempt to offer the mother scraps of his false self and become the mother's *symbiotic therapist* (Searles 1986). In another instance, the child's incompetence may activate narcissistic wounds and depressive nuclei in the mother, or the archaic functioning of the borderline and psychotic child may trigger the mother's psychotic nucleus and reinforce primitive defense mechanisms (splitting, denial, projective identification, expulsion, foreclusion) that nail the child in the assigned role, perpetuating the vicious circle.

Comparison of material from the two therapies in *supervision* or discussion between the therapists makes it possible to take a long view of *the effect that progressive and regressive changes in the mother fostered by the therapeutic relation have on the child and vice versa.* For example, a mother with a rigid character organization registers any movement of the child in the direction of acquiring a personal or gender identity as a traumatic event or a veritable attack that threatens to undo her balance. Or a child with great narcissistic fragility that renders him extremely dependent on the mother may experience as an

---

receives many sensations, is not a part of his mouth and is overwhelmed with unbearable anger and panic at this presumed mutilation.

attack, an imposition, or violence any shift of the mother's—towards decollusion with the tyrannical, possessive, and vengeful aspects of the child and towards identification with mature objects.

From the technical point of view, it is important that the mother's therapist interpret her resistance to loosening control over the child and share with her the traumatic impact of changes in the child, just as the child's therapist must help him face the narcissistic anger he feels the moment he discovers he is not the center of the mother's life. The child is discouraged from sustaining his capable attempts to exploit the mother's sense of guilt in order to remain the center of attention, and encouraged to give up the secondary gains of omnipotence. In the process, the therapist may learn much from the child about his defensive strategy—how the child "has learned to get in and get out of the mined area of the mother's unconscious to safeguard the identity he has succeeded in winning thanks to his own vitality and to the therapy" (Fé d'Ostiani 1987, personal communication). In the stages of mother and child therapy, one may also follow the evolution of their relations with the father and other family members.

Conversations of the child's therapist with the parental couple prior to psychoanalytic breaks make it possible to verify changes in the child, to go further into the evolution and disturbance of the relationship of the parental couple, with particular reference to parental functions,[8] and to assess the effects of changes in the mother and child on the father and

---

8. Cf. the concept of *parentality*—a function of the parent's mind that fosters the child's psychic integration and growth (Di Chiara et al. 1985, Marion 1993). I believe that in cases of serious pathology in the child, only a therapeutic relationship that produces structural change in the parent's psychic organization can foster that parentality.

other members of the family. Finally, comparison and integration of clinical material from the three settings in *supervision* or in discussion between the psychotherapists help to broaden understanding of the *collusions* that obstruct the development of productive analytic relationships and the evolution of a creative and transformative mother–child relationship.

Pathological collusion in family relations and fusion with the family group, that is, with the collective elements (Neri 1993), feed pathological fusion between individual members of the family, inhibiting development of new relationships, and also block the experience of the relation with the therapist both in the transference dimension and in that of new relationships.[9] Pathological collusion in the narcissistic mother–child relationship counters the impossible wish for fusion and control (McDougall 1982), the creation of a potential space for developing an intermediate area of experience in which self and object are separated and differentiated and can communicate (Ferro 1992), and the introduction of new meaningful objects into the external and internal relational world of child and mother. All these factors together interfere with the implementation of parental functions and the child's acceptance of his role as child.

The areas of collusion determine a pathology in the relationship that may or may not be serious: the continuum ranges from

---

9. Therapy with the mother and the parental couple—as confirmation and supplement to what may be inferred from treatment of the child—helps identify and go deeper into aspects of the family pathology that prevent or impede the child's development. I refer to transgenerational fantasms (Lebovici 1988) and the transmission from parent to child of sectors of the mind that are split off, denied, or emptied (Green 1973); of unconscious fantasies that become encysted in the form of transgenerational sediments (Bonaminio et al. 1990); of ego-alien factors (Winnicott 1972); of barely integrated introjects from the parents' unconscious that settle in the child (Searles 1986).

collusions limited to fusional and symbiotic areas that ruin the warp of the relationship, to massive collusions that build up interlocking structures in which mother and child are blocked in fixed roles by means of the projective identification of aspects of the self and not just of internal objects, affects, and conflicts (collusion on depressive, perverse, and psychotic nuclei, *folies à deux*, gridlocked relationships[10]).

When the traumatic impingement on the child's emerging self is so massive as to produce an autistic withdrawal or to prevent an integration of the fragmentary primitive nuclei of the physical and psychic self, I do not believe it is possible to speak of collusion. In less extreme situations, the use that a parent makes of the child to complete his/her own defensive system interferes with the formation in the child of an authentic and separate self and with the identificatory processes that are at the basis of the sense of identity (Gaddini 1969). By identifying with pathological rejecting and aggressive as well as healthy aspects of his parents' personalities, the child manages to construct a false self, and by assuming the role assigned to him by the parents, he becomes the *receptacle* in which the parents project impulses and affects and expel aspects of themselves that they reject, hate, or idealize.[11] In the narcissistic relationship, collusion is supported by the built-in circularity and backed up by the

---

10. Racamier (1992) defines the *gridlock* situation as one in which the two partners, mother and child, are meshed in a relationship marked by intense mutual dependency and forced interaction. The gridlocking, he says, is a way of exerting mutual influence totally without any psychic intermediary.

11. The child can be impinged on by specific unconscious parental fantasies (undigested and indigestible by the child), and by the unconscious demands the parents make on him, so that the child sustains "the collusion that stabilizes the couple." In this fashion "the child is put in a situation where his undergoing the trauma performs a reparative function

mutuality of projective identification and mirror-like experiences.

The reasons for a child's colluding with his mother vary with the type and seriousness of the pathology. The child may not have a sufficiently aggressive drive to grow because of a constitutional ego deficiency or some genetic anomaly. Or the child may be satisfying an omnipotent fantasy of staying fused with the mother as a defense against catastrophic anxiety about separateness, anxieties about his own death and his mother's death, or castration anxieties activated by impact with the oedipal. The child may identify with pathological aspects of the mother's mental functioning and use the same archaic defense mechanisms (denial, splitting, projective identification), so that the relation is one of mutual expulsion and rejection. Perhaps an absent or pathogenic father may be unable to perform the paternal function of helping the child separate from the mother or become a component of the oedipal triangle at a whole-object level, and there may be no alternative figures within the family or outside to whom the child can bring his dependency and relation needs. Or, finally, hate and rancor due to deprivation may prevent the child from accepting any restriction and reparation from the mother.

The collusive mother–child relationship enters into crisis when factors internal to the couple (the emergence of ambivalent drives, the desire of either or both to discover and grow) or external (changes in the family nucleus, school and job demands) upset the functioning of the couple as a self-sufficient unit. In a narcissistic relationship, therapy for only one of the partners could produce a crisis in the other or lead to the interruption of the therapy in the case of the child. Therapy with

---

for the parental couple," at the expense of his own right to exist (Giannakoulas, personal communication).

both mother and child helps to *break up the gridlock of collusion* and *darn the fabric of the relationship* to the extent that each analytic setting fosters construction or reconstruction of the psychic apparatus—of a *mental container* for fantasies, representations, affects, and thoughts—and so reduces the tendency to discharge tension and act out archaic conflicts in the relationship and to use the other as a complement to oneself; in other words, *it reduces the interactive pathology*. Also, in each setting there is a working-through in the transference of the intensely persecutory pathological internal object relationships that are acted out in the mother–child relationship and distort it.

The metaphor of the fabric of relationship, albeit overused, was suggested to me by a child who reported that shortly before coming to his session he and his mother had eaten off a frayed tablecloth that was all spotted and stained. The child's words might have been a reference to the quality of maternal holding and feeding or to anxieties linked with his drives and with conflict in the transference, or they might have been "the communication of the child as the analyst's best colleague in response to what had been exchanged at the previous session" (Ferro 1992, p. 23). Still more appropriate in the context seems the hypothesis that the tablecloth was like a screen on which the mind and thought of mother and child were projected. I associated the holes in the fabric to empty spaces in the psyche where mother and child colluded, which at the level of subjective experience perpetuated the reciprocally mirrored exchange of feelings of emptiness and non-existence and on the level of mental functioning might be defined as areas of non-identity. The torn fragments evoked the laceration of narcissistic wounds which they expected each other to heal. It seemed that the child was asking (and I could not but take account of it) to try out a different kind of relationship with me as a new object and also to reweave the relationship with the mother in the sense of restoring the flow of eutrophic fantasies and introducing a space for play, imagination, thought, and verbal communication.

Family members engaged in parallel therapy find *meaning* as well as *utility* in it. For one thing, the chance to try out a new relationship with the therapist, to experience an object that "takes in transference and proposes relationship" (Ferro 1992b, p. 57) introduces new elements into the mother–child relationship and that of other family members. The therapies of mother and child have a salutary influence on each other if, after both have experienced a relationship with an object that takes in projective identification without its violence, mother and child can relate to each other. The child's therapist may take in the projection of an introject of a witch-mother, say, who imprisons and kills babies (and by whom the child is frightened) but the therapist, unlike the real mother, does not react by becoming the witch the child wants the therapist to become. Similarly, when the mother's therapist takes on the child role he takes in the projection of damaged and rejected parts of the mother's self, but the therapist, unlike the child who becomes the caricature of a rejected turd, does not give them substance. The therapist may thus be introjected as an active container that neither breaks nor is stretched to the point of suppressing its own right to exist.

The experience of an object that offers a model of a mental relationship that does not pass through the acquisition of data but through the acquisition of quality, passion, and patience (Gaburri and Ferro 1988) improves the *affective quality* of the mother–child relationship. Furthermore, the experience of the aspects of the therapeutic situation that introduce differentiation and rule, both of which are fundamental for building the self and differentiating self and object, makes it possible to experience a relationship other than pathological fusion in family relations. The experience of a relationship that generates affects and hitherto *unborn thoughts* introduces into the mother–child relationship the idea of a coupling that may be *creative* and fertile and endowed with great potential for change.

In an indirect way parallel therapy introduces a *transitional* area between mother and child: they have an experience that is similar in some ways, because it is a therapeutic relationship, and dissimilar in others, because the therapy is conducted by different people. The presence of a third party (the other one's therapist) fosters an untraumatic separation of the child from the mother and opens the way for both of them to seek new relationships, the first of them with *the father*, as we shall see in the next chapter.

I have found that children's resistance to therapy is often connected with a sense of guilt, a feeling of betraying mother with a mother–father–friend therapist who is more understanding and invites the child on a voyage (a voyage of the mind) from which the mother and other members of the family are excluded. Parallel treatment of the mother allows the child to trust himself to the analyst and establish a therapeutic alliance without feeling guilty toward the mother.

Some kinds of negative therapeutic reaction may also be interpreted on the basis of a kind of *fidelity* to original objects. I have noticed that they appear when the therapist fails to understand that the child brings not only his traumatized and rejected self but also the damaged objects with which he identifies. I do not mean internal objects damaged by the child's destructiveness, sadism, and greed, but the deprived and disturbed real objects, correctly perceived as such, from which the child cannot separate, not out of guilt but out of intolerable pain and a sense of powerlessness at now being able to treat them. One way of meeting the impasse generated by negative therapeutic reactions of this sort is to offer the parents therapy. I was struck by the sense of relief and gratitude that a mute psychotic child felt and expressed when his mother entered a parallel setting; I might instead have expected possessiveness of the autistic child, a reaction of anger and jealousy because of exclusion. (I can still see the perplexed and conflicted look on the face of a child who fought off his jealousy and went into a session in his therapy room, allowing a new puppy to accompany the mother into hers.[12])

I use the term *parallel*, which I prefer to the term *simultaneous* used by Anna Freud and her school, because I have found that the therapeutic process leading to change in the mother, child, and their relationship, evolves in gradual stages that are reached by mother and child in parallel fashion—therapeutic alliance, transference, the capacity for object relations, triangulation, the ability to play together and to communicate connected with the existence of a transitional area. In the next chapter we shall see that *the creation of a space for play in the child corresponds to the creation of a space for dreams in the mother.* The fact that mother and child have a parallel therapeutic existence does not mean that their own relationship remains unchanged or that the two experiences never touch, which might seem to be the case if we stopped at a literal

---

12. In the analysis of an adult borderline-psychotic I overcame the impasse of a negative therapeutic reaction caused by a sense of guilt because the other family members were left out of the analysis (the others often coinciding with aspects of the patient that attack the analysis), by giving ample room in the analysis to working through family relations. In the case of adults whose parents are dead, some impasses and negative therapeutic reactions have been resolved when the patient perceived my readiness to accept the projection into me of a disturbed parent and to acknowledge his correct perception in me of blind spots. This was the first step that helped me respond to the patient's wish to treat me as an aspect of himself and as other than self.

reading of the term *parallel*, for in fact each of the parties has an affective and cognitive experience that enriches and transforms their own relationship. So that mother and child may discover elements of originality, freedom, uniqueness, and creativity in their relationship, they can separate and come together again on the affective and imaginative plane in that shared mental space where the creativity of the couple finds its origin and expression. Collusion can finally be restored to its etymological roots as "playing together."

7

PARALLEL PSYCHOTHERAPY OF MOTHER AND CHILD IN INFANTILE PSYCHOSIS

In the following therapy excerpts from three cases of child psychosis with language absence,[1] the mother and child couples were followed in parallel but separate settings in the same private service. Edda and Alessio, Giorgia and Bruna, and Anna and Romina were treated once, twice, and three times a week

---

1. The absence of speech is certainly a limitation on the implementation of psychoanalytic psychotherapy, but not on the construction and evolution of a relationship in the pure state, as it were, beyond words. The child moves from autistic closure and rejection of the relationship towards experiencing a relationship that is structuring for the self and the relationship and for the birth of thought. Careful assessment of the child's emotional responses to the therapist's mental processes and the transference and countertransference shifts makes it possible to distinguish progressive movement from regressive movement or impasse. Moreover, careful observation of changes in the child's spatial position and the way he communicates (from cryptic messages conveyed in stereotyped gestures to the expressiveness of preverbal mimic speech) makes it possible to follow the shift from narcissistic (adhesive and projective) to introjective identification.

respectively; in each case, the parental couple met the child's therapist three or four times a year on the occasion of holiday breaks in the analysis. The three children were subjected to several medical and diagnostic examinations and to re-educative intervention.

The three mothers had serious personality disturbances (borderline personality organization, according to Kernberg's 1984 classification) and all were in what Green has termed "the state at the limit of analyzability" (1990). All three mothers, either individually or with spouse, had already experienced supportive psychotherapy from the doctors, psychologists, and professionals to whom they had turned for their children. Romina's mother, Anna, had had group and marital therapy. Bruna's mother, Giorgia, and father had support conversations with their daughter's neuropsychiatrist. Edda, Alessio's mother, at first with her husband and then on her own, had regular meetings with her son's therapist (me) before embarking on her own psychotherapy at the same hour and in the same service where I saw Alessio.

The material here is based on my supervision of the therapists of Romina and her mother, Anna, and Bruna and her mother, Giorgia, and on my own treatment of Alessio and my editing of the notes from his mother's therapist. I subdivide the therapy of the mothers into representative stages and illustrate the parallel evolution in the child's setting and in that of the parental couple.

FIRST STAGE

At the start none of the three mothers has any motivation for personal analysis. The shared refrain is "I only come for my child, in the hope that something can be done to help." Anna's resistance derives from the narcissistic wound of having a child who did not meet the expectations of the dream child, Giorgia's from guilt for having a child who was always rejected, and Edda's from unconscious awareness of her own serious pathology. (Note that a series of deaths and traumas marks the history of two of the mothers, Giorgia and Edda.)

• Bruna, an 8-year-old Down syndrome girl with psychotic symptoms, was born five years after a brother died in an accident he caused himself and after an unsuccessful attempt at adoption. Although Giorgia had not wanted another child, she did not terminate her pregnancy because she wanted "to provide company for her older child and to please her husband"; she was unaware of the gender and the genetic defect of the child in her womb.

• Alessio, a boy with an autistic psychosis, was born shortly after his parents separated. The father left the mother at an advanced stage of her pregnancy after several years of marriage for another woman.

• Romina, a 5-year-old first child, had a form of autism; neonatal brain damage was suspected but never confirmed. She had been fantasized as a "princess from a royal family who was coming into the world in a marvelous home. Everything was so perfect and then the great misfortune." This was the content of a dream the mother (an infantile narcissistic personality) had after two years of therapy.[2]

Insistent requests for advice and reassurance about the child

---

2. It is a well-known concept that the more the mother is on the narcissistic side, the more imperative it is that the child send the mother a gratifying idealized picture of herself. This image is, in fact, necessary for the child's cathexis. Racamier (1992) describes cases in which "one observes the move from the exasperated narcissism of a mother who will never mourn her own ideal illusions to the psychosis of the child or the adult" (p. 68).

characterize this first stage and pose substantial technical problems. The meaning of the requests must be assessed case by case. In general they seem to reveal an infantile and concrete level of dependency and the impossibility of imagining a relationship that might become therapeutic *through the sharing of a psychic reality without changing the objective reality of having a disturbed child*. Sometimes the violence with which advice is sought underlies a fantasy of concrete appropriation of a piece of the omniscient and omnipotent mother.

• Alessio's mother, Edda, had narcissistic personality disorders with borderline functioning. She resisted linking because accepting therapy would have meant accepting a reality that she rejected and that no therapy could ever change: her husband had left her, her son had problems, and she had to work for a living. The therapeutic process could not even start because interpretation, especially transference interpretation, was scorned and ridiculed and everything was brought back to a seeming discourse about reality. The therapist had great difficulty in containing the mother's destructiveness and aggressiveness. In the countertransference she felt Edda's destructiveness like the sensation of having a squid in her head, her brain reduced to ground meat, or a sensation of befogging torpor. At other times when Edda discharged her aggressiveness suddenly, unexpectedly, she had to struggle against the threat that everything that had been built up would be wiped away in one fell swoop. The mother's aggressive manner seemed similar—in its suddenness and unpredictability and its apparent senselessness, as well as in the countertransference response it evoked—to outbursts of aggressiveness that the child acted out in his therapy. In the child's case, these outbursts corresponded to moments of nonintegration or disintegration. Part of Edda's communication was preverbal and acted out, in the sense that Edda did not collaborate by associating, dreaming, or speaking but expressed herself by impersonating aspects of her self and acting out fragments of behavior that produce experiences that are subsequently thought in the countertransference (Bollas 1989).

• Romina's mother, Anna, had an infantile narcissistic personality and used the therapy to discharge complaints about everything and everyone, evoking a sense of impotence and uselessness in the therapist. Later she used the containment to extroflect more directly a violent aggressiveness against herself and her internal and external objects. Anna denigrated the mother who was a slave to her husband, she idealized the rich and powerful father, she devalued her own husband, and repeatedly threatened to break up the family. There was no kind of empathy with her children's needs, especially those of the psychotic daughter. Romina had never existed for her. Romina was not an irreparably damaged object for her but rather "a being from another planet" that Anna could not face, something dangerous to be shunned.

• Bruna's mother, Giorgia, had a depressive masochistic personality structure. From the start, she felt that it was impossible to separate from her daughter and let her go. She experienced separation from the object as a violent tear that caused hemorrhaging (indeed, she had repeated hemorrhages on the occasion of analytic separation). Her ambivalence towards her daughter gave rise to an excited sexual sadistic relationship and to an openly declared impulse to free herself by getting rid of her.

In this first stage all three mothers display psychotic-type resistance that takes the form of attacks on the setting and the analytic function.

SECOND STAGE

The mother begins to accept a therapy for herself. "The experience of a clinical space in which to construct or reconstruct the experience of being contained by the body and psyche of another" (Bollas 1990, p. 16) fosters the emergence of the transference. Even if the mother continues to keep the analyst in the position of object exclusion and to maintain that she does not need her own therapy, she betrays a desire and curiosity to know herself and what is happening in the relationship with the child. The child's problem stops being used as resistance. The disturbed child remains, however, the locus where her own child self is shifted and where psychotic and perverse elements of the mother's personality are projected.

• It was clear in the case of Edda that the child lacked a transforming presence and was forced to act out because his structure was insufficiently mature to contain amounts of the mother's aggressiveness and destructiveness that even the mother's therapist, often in the role of child during therapy, found it hard to contain.[3] In other words Alessio was being asked unconsciously to be the mother's symbiotic therapist, according to the unconscious equation in which the child equals the parent (Searles 1986).

When the psychotic child and the mother's older children appear in dreams, the therapist can take a first step towards putting the mother in touch with the needy and instinctual

---

3. Green (1990) says that "it is the struggle against intense, uncontained drives coming from the object which should be allied and which instead become an enemy that mobilizes the destructive drives responsible for the development of psychosis . . . psychosis would thus be an exorcism of the object . . . it is established when the subject is forced to mobilize his destructive impulse as a way to end the fusional relationship with the early object" (p. 181).

aspects of her own infantile self projected into her son. The mother can be told, thanks to the evidence of the dream, that the psychotic child in the dream is not the *real* psychotic child, but an aspect of her own self that she is able to *represent* in the dream. The mother can also be shown that the other children coincide with healthier aspects of her self or those more narcissistically cathected (Freud 1914).

The mother develops empathic attitudes towards the psychotic child's needs when she feels she can bring her own fragile and traumatized aspects into her own therapy as well as indirectly into her child's therapy, and when she feels that her negative and rebellious aspects and the concrete attacks on the setting, including failure to pay, do not destroy the therapist and the analytic function. In other words, the mother's *parenting* improves to the degree to which she can bring aspects of her *real self* into the therapy. Thanks to identification with the therapist, first imitatively and then introjectively, the mother "learns" to manage the relationship with her son on the basis of "good sense"[4] rather than collusion with perverse and psychotic aspects; to distinguish impulses that should be frustrated from needs to be satisfied; to oppose aggressive and destructive behavior, which must be contained though not violently repressed; and, above all, to protect the libido aspects of the relationship with the child. I believe that a constant disciplined attitude constitutes adequate and transformative holding for both child and parents. When parents are unable to educate the child to frustration, and leave him at the mercy of his destructiveness

---

4. Tustin (1990) notes as important therapeutic factors that foster emergence from autism the therapist's undivided availability and attention, firmness, clarity, and *good sense*. The therapist must want to learn from children and establish an empathic relationship with them, which, however, will not affect the therapist's objectivity and separateness.

and impulses, there are several reasons: fear of the child's anger and of losing his love; terror of the anxiety and vulnerability of the child, who defends himself by hyperactive, tyrannical, and aggressive strategy and behavior; dread that the child will "clam up." In this last case, it is not infrequent that parents insist on overstimulating the child in such a fashion as to oppose those physiological regressions that foster moments of integration.

• Romina's mother "discovered" that if you put out rat poison you risk poisoning dogs. In other words, she discovered that to eliminate the greedy and destructive "mouse" aspects of her daughter, she also killed unconditionally trusting and affectionate living parts.

The mother's relationship with the ill child is now protected because she projects onto her husband and other surrounding figures her own rejection and sadistic impulses towards the child or correctly perceives those same aspects in them. Working through fusional and symbiotic aspects by way of the retrieval of parts of the self that have been split off and projected into the child seems to precede the possibility of looking at the relationship with the husband, into whom scorned and destructive aspects of the self had long been projected, partly in order to maintain an analytic space that was fairly free of conflict.

Therapy with the mothers makes it possible to get back to the personality of the mothers' parents, the disturbance in the relationship of that parental couple, and the way in which the parents influenced their daughters' personalities. By analysis of defenses, anxieties, and fantasies, the therapy fosters the recovery of positive identifications and libido aspects in the relationship with internal and external objects.

The Children's Therapy

The children's therapists worked to provide the containing and transforming presence that all three children had lacked. From a situation initially characterized by autistic withdrawal— an avoiding attitude and obsessive rituals that serve a self-containing function against anxieties of being annihilated in the case of Alessio, serious self-destructive manifestations and stereotyped rocking in Bruna, sensual self-excitement alternating with outbursts of uncontrolled aggressiveness in Romina—the children and the therapists began to experience the relationship. Repeated analyst's interventions, aimed at modulating experience within the therapeutic relationship, made the children eventually begin to develop *preliminaries of thought*. The relationship evolved from one of rejection and narcissistic identification (adhesive and projective identification) to one of introjective identification.

At the beginning it is hard to find the right distance (spatial and emotional) from the child and still stay in touch. In order to maintain or regain emotional touch with the child, the therapist often seeks reassurance in his culture. Her voice can be experienced as a warm bath of words in which the child is wrapped, a warm cover that conveys something embracing and human as against a hard and rejecting not-me, or the voice can be locked out while contact is sustained through touch and sight. In the early stages, words as the vehicle of sense perceptions and even more of emotions may become blunt instruments, violent intrusions that expropriate the self or generate misunderstanding. It is important to find words that can be introjected as vehicles of unambiguous meaning.

The *aggressiveness* of these children arouses painful countertransference reactions, since it touches the deepest roots of the therapist's own aggressiveness. It is important to *decode* the child's aggressive behavior and distinguish between vital and non-vital aggressiveness—aggressiveness that comes from an identification with non-integrated aggressive introjects that belong to the mother's or the father's unconscious (Searles 1986), aggressiveness as defense against persecutory objects and fantasies, and the aggressive drive that arises in the child's own self, constructed as a center responsible for impulses, feelings, and actions.

The concrete aspect of the setting (duration and frequency of sessions) is important to foster the transition from bi-dimensional functioning of the mind to the acquisition of a three-dimensional space in the self and in the object, and the transition from primary anxieties to schizoid-paranoid anxieties and defenses. What is fundamental is to achieve a distinction between self and object, between the inside and the outside of subject and object. Undifferentiated features of the setting—namely the same space, time, and frequency of the sessions—foster the experience of primary fusion with the therapist-setting, equivalent to the mother-environment, which helps to structure the self and provide a sense of continuing existence, whereas discontinuous features of the setting introduce the differentiation of the self from the object and the possibility of internalizing a representation of the absent object in a psychic space.

• For a long time Bruna hit herself violently and rocked at the beginning of therapy; as an alternative to self-destruction she would tear up paper to discharge aggressiveness in a non-neutralized, undifferentiated state. For a long time she rejected the relationship with the therapist and hit herself hard, perhaps to feel that she actually existed. The violent, sensual self-stimulation and negative autoeroticism opposed the cathexis of the object and the introjection of the therapist's function, and attacked the process of symbol formation.

In a second stage Bruna sought an adhesive relationship

with the therapist, positioning her back against the therapist's stomach, turning only briefly for a fleeting glimpse of the therapist. (I have mentioned that Bruna was a Down child who had been rejected during the pregnancy; she was born after the death of a brother, and had never been accepted for what she was but had always been seen and experienced as a concretization of aspects of the mother's and father's selves that they both strongly rejected.) Her self-destructive manifestations became rarer and alternated in the session with masturbation, which was easier to tolerate in the countertransference since it seemed to contain elements of positive libido auteroticism.[5] Sometimes, instead of masturbating, Bruna tried to involve the therapist in an exciting wrestling match on the rug until the midpoint of the session, when she could bear to look at her from a proper distance. Now Bruna could let the therapist see her and she could see herself mirrored in the therapist's eyes.

• Alessio, my patient, moved from an initial position of avoidance and engagement in obsessive rituals, meant to provide self-containment in the face of the anxiety of being annihilated, to one in which he had a kind of remote-control relationship with me, whereby he had me perform actions in his stead, as if I were an extension of him. He would "hook me by eye and ear" and invite me to follow into the chaotic and confused world he reproduced first in the whole office and then in the therapy room by throwing toys, water, and dirt on the floor. There was a long period in which he threw whole and

---

5. Jeammet (1989) contrasts destructive autoeroticism with the positive libido autoeroticism that links experiences of pleasure with the object, which incites reverie (i.e., the pursuit of hallucinatory satisfaction of pleasure) and representation. "The act of reverie," he says, "is a prototype of symbolization and makes it possible to think about the absent object thanks to the quality of the internalizations established" (p. 1767).

broken toys and pieces of wood all around the room (perhaps pieces of the self that were not differentiated from pieces of not-me, bizarre objects). I would gather them up in my skirt or in a basket and arrange them on a table in such a way that they had some sense and a "shared function" (Tustin 1990). Working through catastrophic anxiety linked to the rupture of fusion with the primary object made it possible for Alessio to separate from me and trust that he would find me again.

He achieved the ability to be alone after a long period in which he would go in and out of the therapy room taking turns shutting himself and me outside the room. Stereotypes diminished, and he learned to use his hands to carry objects and his pockets as personal containers. The relationship changed in the sense that he stopped using me as an extension of himself. Nevertheless I felt paralyzed for a long period while he incessantly repeated the same gestures and rituals with only slight variation.[6] The feeling of being immobilized by Alessio's control in an endless, exhausting session decreased as he acquired more capacity to tolerate emptiness and the distance between self and object, and the persecutory quality of the object lessened. After five years of treatment, I was able to organize a game with Alessio using the table top as a little theater where he could reproduce everything I imagined was his world (home, school, garden), using toys that had so long been ignored and whose symbolic meaning was now recognized. In the beginning he

---

6. Some theoretical explanations about the function of ritual and the importance of repetitiveness in therapy in connection with constructing the self (Soavi 1990) helped me to bear the boredom and exasperation and to stay alive and awake. "Through ritual the autistic child tries to ensure both the cohesiveness of the self and a sense of identity-identicalness, keeping the bad parts at bay," and "to maintain the possibility of active functioning in the face of the threat of inertia resulting from autistic withdrawal" (Fè d'Ostiani 1986, unpublished paper).

could not bear to have me be concerned with the toys, which he regarded as rivals of whom he was jealous. Then he gradually identified with me and helped me. Our collaboration, however, was often threatened by his uncontrollable impulse to throw everything on the floor and *rip off the characters' heads*—a clear attack on mentalization and the therapeutic relationship. The affective quality of the relationship changed: the libido side seemed to emerge as control decreased and vice versa.

In the last stage of therapy Alessio lay on the couch towards the end of the session. He listened to me and accepted my invitation to "chat for awhile;" that is, he replied to my questions with gestures and mimicry so rich that they conveyed a great deal of expressiveness. The "bad fox who gave me low blows" disappeared—the image evoked in me by sudden and unexpected aggressive behavior, and due, as suggested by the countertransference, to an element of ego-alien identification (Bonaminio 1990, Winnicott 1972), or to an uninterpreted aggressive introject of the mother's unconscious (Searles 1986)—and became a beautiful fox printed on the fabric of a soft cushion.

Then came the stage of concern for the object: instead of simultaneous expressions of highly incongruous emotions of love and hate, there was an ambivalent sort of relation. That is to say, Alessio now expressed feelings of love and hate towards me in the therapy and towards his grandmother at home, and showed he was sorry when he feared he had hurt us.

• After a period in which Romina's therapist had difficulty keeping her in the therapy room and not running around the whole office, the child established a relationship, faint though it was: she fluctuated between states of high excitement, in which she grasped the therapist's dress and breast, and intense anxiety—anxiety about being emptied (she dropped a rag doll that she carried around as if it were only a rag) and liquefied (she constantly asked to go pee). Romina's aggressive behavior, pulling the therapist's hair and scratching her face, was correctly interpreted as an attempt to find a space in the mother's mind and in the therapist's. Romina's hair pulling also reproduced a way of relating used by her mother, who would pull Romina's hair to wake her up if she overslept or to get a reaction when she seemed to be prey to anxiety. After three years of therapy Romina could express her need for containment, her possessiveness, her jealousy of rivals, and her sadness at the moment of parting. She was the only one of the three children who learned to speak after the end of five years of therapy.

Breaks in Therapy

Breaks in the therapy seriously threatened its progress in the two settings. In an early stage before separation, mother and child attack the dependency on their respective therapists and regress, reestablishing a pathological collusion that proves partly functional in surviving the break period. At an intermediate stage the mother somatizes and acts out, mainly on the child, who is still confused with the mother's self at the level of corporeal and psychic representation; this somatization and acting out express a condensed version of her pathology, for they show how she deals with psychotic or traumatic areas that could not be worked through at a psychic level.

• Bruna's mother had uterine hemorrhages on the occasions of separation from the daughter's therapist in the third year of therapy and from her own therapist in the fourth year, and she associated them with the dramatic experience of being torn and emptied that she felt at Bruna's delayed birth.

• Well into treatment, Alessio was sent by his mother to summer camp and deprived of his therapy. Edda made sure that her son's therapist would be ready to receive him in case anything went wrong at camp, and she continued her own therapy. She could separate from her son at a time when she felt she was still protected—by her own therapy, by a friend, or by her mother, who came to stay because she could not sleep alone. The way she controlled her separation from her son and from her therapy as the summer break approached helped her maintain her balance, because, living alone with her child and perceiving her own fragility, she feared a breakdown. As a result however, she failed to get in touch with the anxieties and mental pain connected with past and recent traumatic experiences and with the experience of her own rejected infantile self: her traumatized self was shifted to the son the moment she pushed him away, while her identification with the traumatizing object was reinforced (Hautmann 1987). Edda had also been sent away from the family at the age of 2 and at school age, but she did not have or recover any unpleasant memory of those periods of separation.

Alessio passed the test of settling in the summer camp, but he did not separate in the sense that his symbiotic link with the mother continued in the form of a collusion that was expressed in his failure to learn to speak. Alessio acquired the ability to represent the absent object in psychic space, but something prevented the birth of the wish to communicate through verbal language, that is, to belong to the world of speaking adults.

• Romina's mother had her fourth child during the Christmas break in the second year of therapy. It is clear that she was acting out the fantasy of recovering an omnipotent fusion with the object, a fantasy that annulled any distinction between self and object, between child self and adult self, and between male and female.

The unthinkable anxieties connected with the traumatic experience of separateness are dramatically experienced in all their intensity in the parallel setting by the child. The child's therapist must often contain both the child's anxieties and those that the mother implodes into him, sometimes shortly before the session; the therapist specializes in working on containment—that is, in offering a containing and transforming presence at the proto-mental and proto-symbolic level of the formation of the self. Anxieties about the fragmentation and dissolution of the self are expressed by flooding the room or throwing things around. The physical containment and bodily care of the child are precursors of mental containment just as much as the concrete aspects of the setting. The therapist synthesizes both functions: bodily care and physical containment together with mental containment. Thus reverie is divided into the different aspects of bodily, affective, and mental reverie. Containing gestures and words (along with the offer of rags, diapers, and handkerchiefs for drying and containing the anxieties of dissolution and liquefaction of the self), and also intervention aimed at altering oral sadism by reducing the intensity of biting and offering substitute objects, provide a model of physical and mental containment that the child can introject.

I observed a kind of *parental acting out* in all three cases on the eve of breaks in the analysis that might be described as pathognomonic in these situations. The parents started looking into the child's brain and teeth the way an adult hypochondriac seeks out damage in his own organs, for a hole or a cavity that proves there is organic damage: echographs, CAT scans, and visits to the dentist were intensified before psychoanalytic breaks. The term *acting out* stresses the force with which the parents turned to doctors and tests involving intrusive instruments and the overdetermined character of this defense mechanism.

In general the hunt for organic damage seems to be equivalent to an attack on the therapy in the sense of an attack on psychic reality, since evidence was sought for an objective fact in which to believe. In particular, subjecting the child to intrusive medical examination before breaks in the analysis may be interpretable—as an unmentalized reaction to being abandoned by the therapist, short-circuited in the relationship with the child (i.e., acted out on the child), who is confused with the self; as a lapse in parental functions, *understood as functions of the mind*, at the moment when the therapist's parental functions are to be interrupted; or as seeking reassurance about the effects of ambivalence and rejection on the child.

But why should reassurance be sought in tests involving instruments that penetrate the body in an intrusive way? Simply because it satisfies the negative pole of ambivalence towards the child or the wish to be free of an early defective relationship by confining it in the child's body (Mancia 1985, Robutti 1992)? Or is it possible that the emotional contact with the phantasy of the primal scene, activated in the mother at the moment of separation from the therapist, is acted out and reproduced in the doctor–child couple, with the mother in the position of the excluded third party who watches and identifies with one or the other member of the couple? Children defend themselves from these sometimes massive impingements on the part of the parents during analytic separation by regressing or by accentuating omnipotent control through tyrannical and aggressive behavior that in any case keeps them at the center of attention and reassures them against the terror of being rejected.

• Alessio was not so sorry when his father and mother decided to have his wisdom tooth extracted under total anesthesia before the summer break because this was one of the few occasions in which he could have both parents look after him. The parents were unable to help him face the operation awake with a dentist friend, because there was a collusion with the child about annihilation, and castration anxieties on the part of persecutory objects projected into the dentist. Yet in play Alessio had begun to trust the dentist-father who helped him face his deprivation.

Analytic separation, however, also fosters maturing change.

• Bruna, the Down syndrome girl, always slept with her mother when her father was on night duty or with both parents, her back against her mother's stomach. She was finally made to sleep by herself before the summer vacation. That happened when the collusion among mother, child, and father about sleeping together was interpreted to the mother and the daughter, and, mainly, when the mother began to identify with the therapist (who left her patients on their own during holidays but kept them in her mind) rather than with the daughter whom she rejected and expelled.

When Bruna began sleeping alone, her self-destructive behavior in the session increased. The therapist was able to link this worsening with the analytic separation and also with her exclusion from the parental couple. Bruna was helped to not turn her anger about exclusion against herself, to tolerate emptiness, to face the storm of emotions and drives released by the parental coupling, and to work through the themes of envy and curiosity about birth. The first night Bruna slept alone in her own room with the door shut, the mother dreamt that Bruna came into the parents' room, went to their bed, and had to be sent back to her own room by her mother. Another dream of the mother's shortly thereafter showed that the loss of the object, previously experienced at the bodily level with the symptom of hemorrhaging, could now be symbolized, and introduced a problem about the relationship with her husband. Giorgia reported that she dreamt she was losing blood. Then she woke up and went to the bathroom in fear of having a hemorrhage but there was nothing. She went back to bed and continued dreaming: "My husband came close and wanted to make love from behind. I turned over, but he wasn't there. I woke up and looked for him and found him outside watering the garden."

THIRD STAGE

The relationship with husband and father is worked through in therapy with the mother and child respectively. The mother brings in for consideration the husband and her problems with him only after she has improved her narcissistic image of herself as a mother by working through the relationship of her child self with primary objects (via the transference) and by better understanding what is happening not only between herself and the child but between herself and her other children. At that point, a space is created within the mother for her husband and marital problems. Features of her current relationship with her husband are focused in the transference. The relationship with the husband is worked through by withdrawing the projection of scorned aspects of the self and the negative pole of ambivalence towards her children and the therapy.

Insofar as a psychic space is created where the mother may represent her husband (i.e., *when the father ceases to be excluded from the mother's cathexis and desire*), and insofar as the third party, the therapist's husband, emerges as a good absent object, the child could begin to express interest in, and a wish for, a relationship with the father, with the therapist's husband, and with the mother's therapist.

Regular meetings of the parental couple with the child's therapist before breaks in the analysis make it possible to see whether changes in the wife (resulting from reduction of confusion, working through penis envy and castration anxiety, and the appearance of reparatory attitudes towards children and husband) are perceived by the husband, and whether the father has changed thanks to empathic identification with the child and to the child's ability to evoke a reparatory parental function in him.

• On two occasions, Alessio's father showed that he could not tolerate the birth of a child and he put Alessio between himself and his wife in order to continue a kind of existence that did not threaten the organization of his personality. But he still could not separate from his wife or child. What emerged was a lack of paternal function when his vicarious maternal function was no longer indispensable. Alessio had long brought to therapy a photograph of himself as a small baby to express narcissistic needs for mirroring, but now he began bringing photographs of his father and himself as an adolescent to display his wish to identify with aspects of the father that he admired and idealized—the way he dressed, his love of nature, and his trips to "desert lands!" Alessio learned to accept his father as he was and make a chink in the wall of rejection that he had always faced. But he still could not put an image of his father together with one of his mother.

• Romina's father was at first very much projected outwards towards his work, but he became increasingly involved in bringing up his children to the degree that his wife acknowledged his protective function and sense of responsibility towards the family. Her rejection of femininity and an ungratifying job, however, kept Romina's mother in a position of extreme competitiveness with her husband.

• Bruna's father paid for her treatment, was personally committed, and accompanied his wife and daughter the long distance to therapy. He had a depressive episode when his wife began to become independent (she obtained a driver's license) and when the daughter's self-destructive behavior decreased and he was no longer needed to control its violence. While Bruna's psychosis had functioned as a poultice to protect her father from serious depression, it also imprisoned him in a state of masochistic, impotent resignation in the face of psychic pain and suffering. With Bruna's increased independence and the growth of the first-born son, who was about to become officially engaged and graduate from college, an affective inhibition appeared in the psychic space of the parental couple. It might be considered a point of arrival and at the same time a starting point for transforming the couple's bond, the point at which Bruna's father could allow himself to tenderly and affectionately offer his wife a peeled chestnut in Bruna's presence around the time the couple were planning their first trip without their children.

Improvement in the child, as measured by a decrease in psychotic and perverse behavior, usually coincides with the appearance of a paternal principle in the child, in the mother, and in the father—with the *internalization of paternal functions* rather than identification with the personal characteristics of the real father. I agree with Chasseguet-Smirgel (1985) in considering paternal functions to be the barrier against incest and the introduction of a mental function regulated by the law of the reality principle and secondary process, and against the regressive tendency to go back to the mother's womb and annihilate the difference between sexes and generations.

Within the analytic relationship, the appearance of the *third element* coincides with the mother's acquisition of a capacity for establishing *a therapeutic alliance with the analytic process*[7]— with her acceptance of the function of interpretation and the broadening of "thinkable" areas. Therapeutic alliance with the analytic process in the mothers I have been speaking of is a goal

---

7. It is not only the analyst and the patient who risk being caught up in an interminable idealized relationship, but the analyst, the patient, and the analytic process itself (Bollas 1990).

reached in advanced stages of therapy. It facilitates the working through of somatization, acting out, and the defensive use of the child in a psychic space in treatment. Dreams and associations with dreams show the route from unthinkable emotions toward the representable and the thinkable, and they indicate the evolution of the relationship and significant structural changes.

• Well on into treatment, Giorgia, the mother who had hemorrhages occasioned by separation from her therapist and her daughter's therapist during the early years, twice dreamt that she went with her cousin, aunt, and friend into a room full of enormous potatoes to buy some zucchini squash. Her doctor (who was actually dead) suggested that she pick three zucchini right off the plant, being careful to cut the plant in such a way that it would continue to grow. This dream, like an earlier one, showed that concrete amputation expressed by hemorrhaging on the occasion of separation had been replaced by the possibility of dreaming and symbolizing the loss. The noble zucchini that replaced the poor potato might have something to do with the *zucca*, a colloquial term in Italian for the head. The doctor who recommended a way of saving the zucchini plant might be seen as the third party who fosters both the working through of anxieties of hate and destructiveness connected with otherness, separateness, and loss of the object, and symbolic reunification, following acceptance of otherness and separation. The development of new ego resources and depressive feelings made it possible for Giorgia to mourn her dead parents, her dead son, and her imaginary child.

• In the tenth year of her son's therapy Edda dreamt that she removed her high heels and put on a pair of walking shoes, which faced her with the prospect of being independent and free. Her self was still quite fragile, yet Edda could imagine an independent future and an end to treatment.

• Alessio came to his session with new shoes, polish, and a

brush, expressing his wish to be free, independent, and clean. I understood him to be communicating, by way of several play sequences, that he still needed a mother; that he was struggling against the regressive narcissistic tendency and the temptation to settle into the condition of a poor rejected baby and that he felt dirty because he got excited whenever he slept in the same bed with his mother.

Some collusive aspects of the mother–son relationship surfaced in a session that took place at the time the Gulf War broke out.

• My colleague and I received Edda and Alessio in the waiting room, and it was very clear that the mother induced her son's "rebellious and disruptive" behavior. She maintained an observing ego and showed that she wanted the sequence to be grasped by the therapists, its function being to attract attention and at the same time to discharge unbearable tensions by way of her son.

She told me and her therapist that Alessio was again putting his shoes in excrement. In her session she took the part of the tyrant, rationalizing her position in several ways. She attacked the treatment and ridiculed dreams (she did not at that time remember her dreams) in the "violent and perverse" way that so many times early on had strained the therapist's capacity for thinking. After the session in the waiting room she turned to me in the presence of her therapist and expressed concern that "she had upset her therapist."

Alessio, in his simultaneous session, scrawled the black circles he had long since learned to draw and at the same time made a move to get me dirty. I interpreted this gesture as an irrepressible impulse to dirty the babies he imagined inside me, of whom he was terribly jealous, but also decoded it as an angry request for containment and defense against the tensions his mother imploded and the behavior she induced in him. This request for containment was soon expressed tenderly by his gesture of cupping his hands as if to invite me to go out and buy other "boxes." In the same session Alessio led me to understand, by miming a sexual advance towards me, that he had slept with his mother and been excited. I thought the war news had resonated in the psychotic nuclei of mother and son and that the eroticization had functioned as an organizer, binding excitement and fear together for both of them. (There were also incestuous elements in the mother–son relationship, and they were worked through in the respective settings.)

At this point questions arose about the progress that Alessio might still make. He had learned to protect the relationship with the object and had benefited from the "congruent," healthy, narcissistic cathexis that his therapist and his mother had developed in him, which was demonstrated by his pleasure in wearing nice new clothes and his pride in displaying the medal he won for horsemanship. Moreover, the cohesion of his body self and his balance were a genuine achievement. And he showed a capacity for reparative work in school, where he did practical exercises and helped needy children.

The way Alessio dealt with some kinds of desk work gave me hope that he was about to acquire mental functions that presupposed greater integration of his psychic apparatus and, perhaps, an understanding of the difference between authentic reparation and manic reparation of the self and the object. He stapled cards together instead of arranging them to form a figure or lining them up to make a sequence. Immediately afterwards he gave me a perplexed look because the pretty cards were not in the right place and had staple holes in them. The way he looked at me evoked a sad thought, a doubt, perhaps the same doubt that tormented him and his mother. I wondered with sadness if his primitive mental processes had been irreversibly damaged by the early traumatic relationship with primary objects (early traumatic experience and awareness of the not-me [Tustin 1981]), or if his ego incompetence and cognitive deficit were the result of a genetic disorder. Both hypotheses precluded the possibility that resolution of fusional and symbiotic aspects of the mother–son relationship could give rise to processes leading to the acquisition of speech and reparation of the trauma connected with all the emotions the child felt in witnessing discourse between his parents, exposing him to the feeling of exclusion (Meltzer 1973).

I often wondered how Alessio might have experienced exclusion from the relationship between parents who were separated and spoke chiefly on the telephone, and the relationship between a mother and grandmother who spoke a foreign language. I began to wonder now how I could have him try out in the therapeutic relationship a "dosed" exclusion from the dialogue between me and my good objects, which might mutate into curiosity and a desire to learn to speak.

The mother's shoe dream introduced the idea of ending the treatment, and that prospect fostered a heightened drive for understanding and reparation in both therapeutic relationships. In both settings the collusion between mother and son that had long obstructed the evolution of the treatment process was worked through. Alessio listened quietly when I invited him to grow, look for a job, try to meet girls, wear clean shoes so he would not be rejected like the toy pig we played with, and try to say a few words—why not—with the speech therapist. The mother looked for answers that would extend her understanding of everything that happened, now and in the past, between her and her son and the dog, and between her, her parents, and her ex-husband. She brought in dreams that showed how close she was to understanding that she had used her son as a transitional object (Giovacchini 1986) to release inner tension, to calm herself, to maintain through her son a delicate bond with the outer world, and to express her resentment against her husband and attack him. What was important now was to support her against overwhelming guilt feelings so that she could resolve the overcompensatory factor in her symbiosis with her son.

Would the narcissistic satisfaction of a more cohesive self and the change in the representation of the self, more closely resembling the ideal self, and the internalization of the analyst's reparatory parental function be sufficient for her to give new birth to her son and to herself in a separate existence?

Is it correct to think that the acquisition of speech was obstructed by pathological collusion? It might be better to put the accent on the fact that *collusion in the preverbal area*, the cathexis of mime and gesture language, was supported by vital libido aspects of relationship. It might have represented an attempt to recover the affective dimension of the relationship and the ability to understand each other without words. Also, it protected mother and son from the fear that the child's learning to speak might have upset that balance of survival that had spared both of them the risk of catastrophic separation, in the absence of an object and an environment able to contain unthinkable and unlivable anxieties.

What kind of psychic transformation in the mother, as well as in the child, *would correspond to the child's learning to speak?*

8

THE FUNCTION OF THE THIRD TERM IN THE IDENTITY FORMATION AND SYMBOLIZATION PROCESSES IN CHILD AUTISM

Conducting therapy with psychotic children and their parents has enhanced my understanding of the early stages of the child's formation of self and identity as well as of disturbances of identity (false self) and defects in symbolic functioning in the parents. The birth of the feeling of identity is a rich and complex phenomenon. It is impossible to speak of the early identity-forming processes of a child without taking account of the role of real objects and the traumatic impingement of the parents' unconscious fantasies, and of the defensive and likewise traumatic use that mother or father or parental couple make of the child at the moment his presence begins to threaten the precarious stability of the defensive narcissistic organization of one parent or the other or the fragile equilibrium of the parental couple.

Several considerations confirm my idea that the parents of psychotic children also need psychotherapy. The presence of potentially psychopathogenic factors in the parents is widely marked in the literature and verified by my own experience—

factors arising from traumatic events of the past and vicissi-
tudes of conflicts as well as those inherent in pathological mental
structure and functioning (Ledoux 1984). It is my conviction
that it is important to help the parents out of a situation of
emotional discomfort and confusion by offering them the chance
to play an active and reparatory role in the child's growth
processes.

This chapter is concerned with the relationship constructed
between the autistic child who does not speak and his therapist,
and with the therapist's parental functions (understood as
functions of the mind) that foster change and growth in the
child (together with the affective experience of the therapeutic
relationship). I mean to show that the child's experience of the
setting and the symbolizing structure of the therapist's mind
(the two aspects that configure the treatment situation), by
itself—independent of changes in the environment obtained by
involving one or both parents in a parallel setting—fosters the
process that leads to the structuring of the self, the birth of a
sense of identity, and the possibility of using the symbolic
function.

From the outset, the autistic child is faced with a setting that
jeopardizes the two-dimensional functioning of his mind by
opposing the illusion of fusion with the mother in a world where
nothing begins and nothing ends. (The symbolizing function of
the setting is well known: "the setting . . . [is] the third term
that together with the psychoanalyst and the patient configure a
symbolic and symbolizing structure that functions with three
terms" [Gibeault 1989, p. 1575]). The child also confronts the
three-dimensional function of the therapist's mind, which contains
the double maternal and paternal referent; the child experiences
a relationship with a therapist who performs maternal and
paternal functions in harmonious interaction or alternatively.

The maternal holding and mirroring function allows the

child to experience a continuity of the self, to achieve a state of narcissistic integration and a sense of identity by way of primary or narcissistic identifications. The paternal function—the third term in the analyst's mind—is one of *symbolic mediation*[1] of the fusional relationship in the direction of acceptance of otherness, construction of a separate self, conquest of a psychic space, and psychic activity.[2] In the therapeutic relationship the third term introduces a structuring discontinuity of presence and a modulation of emotional and spatial distance; it endows the relationship with depth and a temporal quality of process that foster the abandonment of adhesive relationship modes and the beginning of symbolization. The need to acknowledge and maintain a distance between self and object is what triggers the process of symbolization.

---

1. What I want to stress with the word "symbolic" is that every move towards separation from the object is accompanied by an operation that symbolizes union at the imaginative and representative levels, first in the transitional area—the intermediate area of experience—and then in the psychic space that is formed in the child as intermediate psychic area (the metapsychic equivalent of intermediate area of experience), which contains the representation of the object and the link with it.

2. I believe that the premises for symbolization are in the link with the mother in the period preceding the separation of me from not-me, in the process through which the mother transforms the data of the child's body into integrated mental images, and in the transitional area. The next step in the symbolization process, leading to internalization of the link with the mother and to the ability to represent the absent object, presupposes the working through of anxieties, hate, and destructiveness connected with otherness, separation, and the loss of the object. Symbolization as an operation implying simultaneous awareness of what links and what separates the symbolized object and its symbol presupposes that otherness and separateness have been accepted and that "there exists in the subject a sufficiently differentiated organization: differentiation among agencies, among images, between inside and outside, between conscious and unconscious, and between the different ways of functioning" (Jeammet 1989, p. 1770).

What I mean by symbolization in this specific context is the ability to think about the absent object thanks to the creation of a psychic space that contains the representation of the object and the internalization of the link with it; the possibility of symbolic play; the ability to communicate anxieties, experience, and conflict through speech and mimicry; and the capacity to use language to facilitate communication rather than block it (as in the cases of barrier-language and ecolalia). The choice of these parameters to indicate the difficult path the autistic child must traverse to reach emotion, thought, meaning, and symbol formation was suggested to me by clinical experience and by Gibeault's definition of symbolization in therapy: "the result of a process that presupposes both the ability to represent an absent object and a subject capable of knowing that the symbol is not the object symbolized" (Gibeault 1989, p. 1574).[3]

The path to symbolization, which the child analyst must traverse together with the mute autistic child, is long and arduous. The analyst's own ability to think symbolically is put to a stern test. It is difficult to create conditions that can introduce sense into the chaos of early traumatic experiences, foster evolution from the bodily to the mental, catch the seeds of rudimentary thought, and promote exchange at the mental level, when the child's needs for physical containment and bodily attention must be seen to, and when the therapist is immersed in the confused, chaotic, and bizarre world the child tries to reproduce in the therapy room.

---

3. Tustin, in treating autistic children, outlines three stages in the development of the ability to use symbols: (1) the phase of "as if" or symbolic equations, (2) the phase of representation by images, (3) the phase of symbolic representation in which the symbol is different from the object to be represented (as the word "cat" does not represent the form of a cat the way a pictogram might).

The first step in dealing with a child who rejects the not-me by using self-protective maneuvers or who tries to cancel any trace of the object by recourse to stereotypes and destructive, anti-introjective, and anti-thought behavior is to foster a relationship by finding a way of *staying together* in the relationship. For example:

- suggesting a proper distance to a child who tries to stick or cling;
- discouraging the use of autistic forms and objects that produce tactile sensation, and fostering the construction of a self by differentiating and integrating opposite sensations (tactile, visual, olfactory, and taste);
- blocking self-destructive behavior with containing gestures and speech before interpretation;
- mirroring and containing the child with one's eyes when the child shuns eye contact or does not look because he has never been looked at for what he is but is seen only as the concrete realization of aspects of the parental unconscious;
- gradually withdrawing from being used by a child as a remote-controlled object in his attempt to avoid awareness of bodily separation and later to omnipotently control the object that he begins to perceive as separate from self;
- remaining awake despite the torpor induced by repetitive and monotonous behavior that becomes veritable rituals.

By analyzing the countertransference the therapist tries to give a name to the anxiety underlying the child's defensive attitudes and behavior, to decode the aggressive behavior, and to trace features of the primary environment and the primary object (one that did not allow the child to have a separate existence, or an intrusive object).

Unlike the real mother, who has no room in her mind for a representation of the child and yet conversely lets herself be completely invaded by the child, the therapist at the beginning offers a *limited space* (the therapy room); the therapist thus implicitly communicates to the child that she is offering him a containing but bounded space in her mind. The subsequent addition of possible therapy spaces comes to coincide with the opening of *new spaces* in the child's mind and in the therapist's and of new spaces in their relationship.

In my experience the transition from the concrete to the mental coincides with the gradual shift from bathroom to therapy room. The child constructs his sensorial self and his bodily identity in the bathroom, thanks to the therapist's "positivizing" work and the therapist's capacity to withstand the pathological and autistic use the child makes of sensorial self-stimulation (production of sensorial shapes, excessive concentration on bodily sensations). The therapist, instead, fosters the evolution and integration of sensations and sensory reactions. The actions, attitudes, and behavior of the child in the bathroom may have the following meanings, depending on the specific situation:

- defense against anxieties linked with the discovery of the object (catastrophic anxieties);
- defense against anxieties linked with the child's acknowledgment of its need of the object;
- association with progressive stages of psychophysical development (acquisition of sphincter control, cleanliness).

Excerpts of clinical material from one child's therapy will demonstrate how mute autistic children become capable of symbolization.

It took a great deal of time and patience to understand that when Alessio provokingly plugged the toilet bowl with a rag he was trying to control the anxiety, activated by the running water, that he might be flushed away with his feces or lose part of his body and the object confused with it. It was only much later that the flush handle became the "good plumber father" who restores the circulation of emotions, fantasies, and thoughts in the mother, blocked by the child's projective identifications.

When he first learned or agreed to turn the faucet on and off by himself, after a long period during which he let the water flood the bathroom, he was showing that he had acquired proper instruments for regulating the flow of excitement and violent sensations. Later he showed that he had learned to regulate his bodily orifices, which were no longer felt to be merely holes left by the rupture of bodily continuity with his object. Regulation of bodily orifices at this point expressed "restored commerce with the object." "It is a matter of transforming bad experiences so that the child can feel that his body has a living inside, that his holes are devices for controlling what comes in and goes out of his body. This is a constituent experience of anal eroticism, since it sets up a dialectic of saving and losing: a true metaphorization of the stomach and the spirit, where the body acquires a psychic dimension and the psyche a physical incarnation" (Gibeault 1989, p. 1584).

Leaving the "unthinking" bathroom and moving to the "thinking" therapy room, a move encouraged but not imposed by the therapist, marked an important shift in terms of wanting to stay in the relationship and the development of mental functioning.

The objects in the therapy room and the play material may be used idiosyncratically. When the therapist follows his intuition and good sense and tries to propose a use according to a "shared function" (Tustin 1977), he is actually choosing objects that have a symbolic meaning and that he believes may subsequently have such meaning for the child as well. For example, the basket may become the therapist's mental womb holding the child together when he feels that he is all in pieces; the boxes may serve to contain and divide good objects from bad—that is, to foster the process of splitting and idealization; the scissors may take the place of teeth for cutting in the making of useful things; the ball may become a concrete object in which the child will project an image of himself, initially still strictly linked to the perception of bodily cavities within (oral gastric cavity), and which only much later will be represented in the drawing of a circle (Gaddini 1959).

Certain sequences of action, activities, and play show the child's access to symbolic functioning in that they contain a *triangular reference*.

Certain interventions of the therapist tend to foster expansion of the symbolic area.

The child acquires the *capacity to be alone*[4] by way of some sequences of trial actions, which he invents when he is trying to control the displeasure and anxieties connected with the loss of the object and which become veritable games when they presuppose the beginning of symbolic functioning.

Alessio slammed the door open and shut, locking out himself and then the therapist, and then he tried to stay alone in the

---

4. The ability to be alone, doing without the real presence of the mother, presupposes an awareness of the continuing existence of a reliable mother and the establishment of an internal environment, which is something more primitive than the phenomenon designated by the term introjected mother (Winnicott 1958).

room or in the bathroom for a few seconds at a time and then longer until he could stay by himself for even minutes at a time. In this period he was able to stay home alone thanks to the fact that the therapist, unlike the mother, could bear the worry of "what is the child doing in the next room or in the bathroom."

The *mirror game* is important for integrating the bodily image of the self, for grasping the difference between a fragmented perception and a unified image of the body.[5] I noticed that the child accepted and enjoyed looking at himself in the mirror only when he could accept the mirror as a substitute for mother's look. The mirror may also contain a reference to a third element, since the child uses it to reflect *the separate images of himself and the mother who are looking in it together.*

After some time, thanks to the mirroring of the therapist and the recovery of the libido cathexis from real objects, the child achieves a cohesive self (libido as the cement of affects).

For months Alessio brought a photo of himself when he was small and kissed it before the start of the session in the presence of his mother and his mother's therapist and afterwards during his session as well.

Better integration of the self provides support for early ego functioning. The pronoun "I," whether the child can utter the word or only points to himself, shows that he has achieved an identity by integrating his bodily image of himself with his "first

---

5. Lacan (1949) writes that in the mirror stage, the infant sees its own image in the mirror as a whole and this perception causes, by contrast, the perception of its own body as divided and fragmented. The ego is the result of identifying with one's own specular image.

introjections and identifications" (Gaddini 1969a), while the appearance of the word "no"—which in the relationship coincides with the constancy of the object—introduces difference, rebellion, and the wish to be separate.

The placement of objects in the therapy room changes with time. At different times one section of the room is preferred over another. The therapist replaces play material; broken toys are thrown away at a certain point the way old things are usually thrown away at home. All these changes are suggested by the *therapist's preconscious* on the basis of messages received from the child, and tend to enhance whatever may favor the development of the capacity for illusion and representation through play.

> I suggested that Alessio pretend the therapy room was divided in two: on one side his bedroom with his cot and table, and on the other the drawing room where I did my work and where we often did things together. He followed my lead and enacted bed time and his anxiety about falling asleep by repeatedly rubbing an eraser on the wall by the bed. I thought it might have been an auditory hallucination, but instead he might have been telling me that he was erasing the bad ugly witch—the not-me aspect of the mother or the father in the primal scene (Gaddini 1974), which he experienced as the witch who wanted to destroy and castrate him.

Telling fairy tales is an extremely important activity and requires that the therapist use the filter of his preconscious functioning in organizing sequences that take on meaning for the child and reflect the child's new ability to introject and project. The therapist takes cards or drawings from books of fairy tales and develops stories based on these stimulus images. Characters are chosen who are meaningful because of their function and role, with which the child can identify himself or the therapist—for example, a doctor, a plumber, a garbage man, a policeman. It is hard for a child to follow a story if he cannot see the image on which it is based and if he cannot identify with the characters who appear. The "triangular reference" offered by this kind of activity is clear, since the child not only pays attention to the sound-music of the therapist's voice but also listens to the *narrative constructions*, which may now be considered as forms of interpretation, since they foster insight.

The wish to build something with the therapist, which shows a drive towards integration and incipient mental activity—both sustained by libido contact with the therapist—is repeatedly threatened by sudden impulses to destroy everything and remains so until the child identifies with the therapist and learns to contain himself alone.

Alessio increasingly managed to keep from ripping off the head of the characters. I interpreted this change as the achievement of a capacity to differentiate himself from an unintegrated aggressive introject from the mother's unconscious that attacks mentalization and with which the child defensively identified (Searles 1986).

When the child agrees to share with the therapist interest in a third element—that is, when he is willing for the therapist to pay attention to something or someone other than him—the child begins to *play*, both in the sense that a space for play has been made in the transitional area and in the sense that the child can use toys to represent his inner and outer world and to communicate with the therapist.

Though Alessio did not know how to play nor did he have the ability to "personify" in the Kleinian sense (Klein 1929), he could somehow dramatize his effort to live, his struggle against a tendency towards narcissistic regression, and his wish to find the object again after having lost it and destroyed it. This might be the beginning of symbolization in Segal's (1957) sense—symbolization as the ability to feel the loss of the object and the wish to recreate it inside the self.

Gesture and mimicry and the ability to express emotions that precede the use of verbal language in some cases become a veritable *preverbal mimic language*. I think that this may be considered a symbolic form of communication in the sense that an internal language seems to be developed, and the child's private language (representation through play, internal language) evolves in the sense of becoming a language for communicating (Giannotti and De Astis 1986).[6]

The acquisition of verbal language shows that the internal mental activity of verbalization, understood as the formation of an internal meaningful language, has been enriched by the additional capacity for vocalization, that is, externalizing the acquired linguistic competence and communicating verbally with an object that is now perceived as other than self. The development of verbal language also shows that therapy has fostered the process of integrating thing presentations and word representations and the transition from visual thought of an imitative kind to verbal thought of a symbolic kind (Gaddini 1969b, Giannotti

---

6. Giannotti and De Astis (1986) maintain that the child's early communications, and also speech, continue for some time to have an essentially concrete and hence bodily value for the child. Only through the organization of an affective relationship can speech attain the level of representation and thus allow the passage to symbolization.

and Del Pidio 1991). Also, there has been a change in the quality of the relationship with the mother (who is in parallel therapy), and the component of active refusal of the child to learn to speak has been overcome. This advance, depending on the specific case, may be due to an attempt to avoid the already-occurred catastrophe of traumatic separation from the mother, to fear of losing one's own contents through speech, to control of oral-sadistic and anal-sadistic drives towards the object, to overcoming mistrust of speech as a highly ambiguous instrument.

Geometric drawings by autistic children do not have symbolic value according to Balcone and Giannini (1987). But I believe that if this kind of drawing is evaluated in relation to the evolution of the transference and the countertransference, it may represent a moment of reflection, of effort towards knowledge of corporal and emotional experiences that until that point were only acted out.

Drawing might also be a sublimation of libido drives, since the child shows he wishes to please the therapist and enter into a loving union with the therapist by offering the drawing.

Alessio reproduced his drawing of a circle with different forms, numbers, and spacing on the page and seemed to express in turn a representation of himself as separate; a representation of positive and negative hallucinatory images based on vague memories of perceptions inside his body— by filling the circle with black he seemed to want to represent anxiety about detachment and that which was lacking, while by drawing an un-dirtied circle several times on the page he seemed to wish to give a positive quality to the hallucinatory image of a breast that fills or of the oral and gastric cavity which are filled; an abstract representation of a mental experience of nonexistence and emptiness.

The mat, the equivalent of the couch for the adults, is used in a later stage of therapy and for varying lengths of time during the session, when the child can relax and get in touch with his state of mind and feelings. He may use it to communicate his temptation to act out his impulses and his excitement, or, lying down quietly, he may think about absent objects, that is, reactivate the memory of gratifying experiences linked with them, relive the moment of separation without anxiety, and anticipate and postpone the moment of future encounter. The memory of the object is full of affective contents (Gaburri 1993). Trust in the constancy and love of the object gave Alessio the capacity to be alone and to experience the absence of the object. It is in the locus of the absence that the capacity for forming and using symbols and experiencing the solitude that is necessary to love the object and to feel the object's love originates (DeRisio 1996). Alessio made it clear that he left his dog in the car before coming to the session. He smiled because he knew he would not forget to go get the dog and that the dog trustingly waited for him.

Interpretation is no longer felt as a third object containing all the hard and bad aspects of the mother and all the negative feelings of the child but rather as something desirable that fosters insight and growth. The possibility of staying together in silence shows that there is now depth in the relationship and psychic space has been won. The child may have a good fusional experience with the therapist when the sense of narcissistic wholeness and identity is sufficiently consolidated so that the presence of the object is not felt to be dangerous and threatening; when the Yes that followed the No that introduced difference and rebellion becomes a Yes that means real affirmation, agreement, and acknowledgment of similarity in a context of difference.

The foregoing describes some therapeutic interventions aimed at fostering cognitive and affective symbolization through the modulated presentation of the third object.

What follows outlines the evolution of the third object as it is perceived and recognized by the child during the course of therapy. From the child's point of view, the third object develops along a continuum going from the perception of a hard and threatening not-me (the end of the session that makes the child totter, the telephone that pokes a hole in the ears, the edge that wounds)[7] and of a *not-mother not-me* (an essential third element in the mother's mind that refers to the presence of thoughts about the father, her own or the child's, and in the child's mind to the recognition of a third party who gradually becomes distinct from the mother in the primal scene), to *a positively defined third object*—the third object containing the therapist mother; the third object that fosters separation, development, and growth in opposition to the wish for narcissistic regression and rejection of reality; the third object that regulates the exchange of communication between mother and child by blocking crossed projective identifications that establish areas of collusion and symbiotic nodes. The third object also takes the form of superego demand that establishes a barrier to incest and introduces mental functioning regulated by laws of secondary process against the regressive tendency to go back to the mother's womb and annul the differences between sexes and generations (Chasseguet-Smirgel 1985).

In the child's psychic space the image of the therapist's husband comes to life when the child perceives him—and the therapist presents him in play and in interpretation—not only as a possible repository of paternal functions and superego

---

7. Any sharp-edged form or object plunges the child into awareness of three dimensionality and physical separateness. Thus, squares and triangles and any other angular form are avoided (Tustin 1990).

demands or as an accessory figure in bringing up children but as *an object of the mother-therapist's desire*. This is a new experience for psychotic children whose parents seem to be two ships that pass in the night without ever meeting.

> Alessio slapped his own hand when he was tempted to pull my necklace or grab my skirt. He thus communicated the fact that he had internalized the incest taboo, a taboo that did not come solely from a paternal demand present in the mother-therapist but also from the image of a father, the therapist's husband, whose existence was mentioned in session and towards whom the child began to show interest, curiosity, jealousy, and rivalry.

It seems important in this phase that the child experience exclusion from the verbal dialogue he imagines between the therapist and the therapist's husband-father, not as a catastrophic void or a violent and threatening primal scene but as an emotional and drive event that could result in a wish to communicate at the verbal level and one day mate the way grown-ups do.[8]

---

8. Gaburri suggests that the experience of exclusion-inclusion from the primal scene might be a third step after encounter-dialogue with the mother's mind (which contains and transforms the child's anxieties about death), and acquisition of the ability to work through the absence of the concrete object. He says that this third experience might be considered "a completion of the link between mental language and speech, introducing a new paradigm that considers discourse between parents as an equivalent of the primal scene" (Gaburri 1993, p. 88). Gaburri's idea supports my contention that the psychotic child who does not speak, but who has acquired "the ability to represent the absent object and to know that the symbol is not the object symbolized" and who has acquired inner language, *does not succeed in transforming feelings of exclusion from the "verbal" primal scene into a desire to belong to the world of grown ups who speak.*

Autistic children have taught me that even in personality structures marked by extreme adhesive identification, the desire to be separate is never totally absent, and separation anxiety is never disassociated from the wish to separate—nor is the wish ever absent to enlarge the network of affective and social interaction and to think. Indeed, thinking and significant relationships would save the autistic child from endlessly mirroring depressive and nonexistence experiences back and forth with the mother. Thanks to the possibility of constant reference to a third element, the therapist becomes the guarantor of these wishes where father, mother, child, and environment have all failed.

9

FROM THERAPY
OF THE CHILD
TO THERAPY
OF THE PARENTS

Why do parents decide to undergo psychotherapy parallel to that of the child on the model I have proposed—in separate settings, with therapists who are in contact with one another—instead of their own psychotherapy (marital or individual) or that of the child?

Based on my experience, I see three models for choice. In the first case, parents need an identification model that allows them to improve their parental role; the more the child's therapist takes charge of the child's pathology and the more the parents' therapist develops and sustains the parents' functions, the more the child improves. In the second case, parents are unconsciously aware of their own pathology and, therefore, potentially motivated towards personal analysis; the child's disorder puts the parents in touch with their own personal distress, and thus, offers them the opportunity to start personal therapy. Psychotherapies take place separately, parents and child each following his own therapeutic course. In the third case, parallel therapy satisfies the parents' fantasy of controlling the child and their relationship with him.

Parallel therapy presented as a multiple setting and including an exchange of information between the different therapists seems to me to be the only alternative to family therapy that can be accepted by parents who are fused and confused with their child and cannot surrender intrusive and controlling ways of relating with him (or by children who cannot face personal therapy because they have difficulty in establishing a relationship with people outside the family). In fact, parallel therapy is seen as a proposal that initially respects the degree of fusion, pathological or not, present in the parent–child relationship. At the same time, it satisfies the desires of both to experiment with new situations and new relationships, without feeling guilty towards one another. The processes of mourning, loss, and renunciation of possession, which lead to separation and individuation in the child and parents, can undergo parallel elaboration in the respective settings.

When treating mothers with a narcissistic pathology, one can see how the child, whose role is to complete the mother's identity and maintain her defensive narcissistic organization, is allowed to separate as the mother's therapist takes charge of the anxieties that up to then had to be managed within the mother–child relationship. This is the first step towards acceptance of the treatment relationship, which eventually leads to structural changes in the mother's personality. As good dependency on the therapist develops, there is a reduction in the tendency to achieve a self-sufficient unit with the child. The mother's therapy evolves to foster narcissistic restoration, the change from narcissistic to introjective identifications, the restoration of the symbolic function, and the integration of depression. The elaboration of collusions in the setting of the child and that of the couple, as well as the birth of ambivalence as the dividing force in both the child and the mother, are important advances towards separation and individuation and towards object relationship.

My direct and supervisory experience with parallel therapy is *a model* that, integrated with countless other models offered by modern psychoanalysis, has facilitated my approach to those clinical situations (not necessarily serious pathologies) in which account must be taken of *current* family relations in which archaic conflict, mourning, and traumas that cannot be worked through intrapsychically are managed by a play of rigid interaction. I seem to have an extra chance when, in consultation or in therapy, I am faced with parents who have structural deficits (identity disorders, false self, areas of non-identity) or disorders in mental functioning (lacunae of the symbolization process) that interfere with the parental function. I am thinking of mothers in analysis who talk about their children all the time, adults who tend to act out primarily on their children, and parents of adolescents with serious pathologies (drug addiction, anorexia, antisocial behavior, psychosis) who refuse therapy.

This last is the case of the woman in question, a mother who asked me for a consultation for her adolescent son, a mother like many others who turns to the therapist as a last resort, crushed by the failure of the many manipulations she has tried in order to adapt reality to the son's pathology. Psychotherapy initiated two years earlier by the son, and which "could have been a solution," had been interrupted after less than a year. I have chosen to use this clinical situation, therapy with the mother of a borderline adolescent, to show how, after a long period of preparation needed to motivate the mother to have treatment, it was possible to impact therapeutically on the child via the mother, at least in part, until the child decided to enter therapy himself with a new psychotherapist two years after the mother began.

The mother's treatment produced a restructuring of all the

family relations and a redistribution of anxieties, as well as an elaboration of her relationship with her son. During the mother's second year of therapy, the son had a psychotic breakdown followed by a prolonged episode of psychotic regression; these events provided an opportunity, so to speak, for the parents to painfully acknowledge their son's fragility and need for care, also a chance for the son to integrate into a new image of himself aspects that would have remained split and unelaborated and to access the individuation processes and the structural maturational changes of adolescence.

Laura asked for a consultation to talk about the problems of her 16-year-old son Antonio. The first time she came alone, the second with her husband. Antonio had begun psychotherapy, twice a week with a psychoanalyst expert in treating adolescents, because for some time he had had a student's block and then became "worried and depressed." But therapy was suspended after less than a year because he skipped sessions and acted out away from treatment, although the mother had "had him escorted to his sessions and was in frequent telephone contact with his therapist." (Mother–child collusion put an end to the treatment.) During an interview with the mother, the son's therapist had thought it advisable to inform her that Antonio was at serious risk because, aside from taking drugs, he was involved in dangerous illegal trafficking. Since the boy refused to go back to his therapist or try any other type of psychological approach, the mother expected me to give her "support to help her son."

When Antonio's parents came together to the second interview, I was faced with a parental couple that Bollas would define as *normotic* and McDougall would call *normotype*, two active and intelligent people whose intellectual vivacity came at the expense of internal reality. The mother talked incessantly, without stopping; the father listened without taking part. Both showed aversion, fear, and disorientation towards a psychological rather than practical approach to problems. After a certain number of interviews, the father declined to participate while the mother continued to come alone, according to the agreed-upon schedule of one session every fifteen days. As the mother spoke about her son, a character came to life inside her who was presented to me in this fashion: "Antonio is a nice intelligent boy who has stopped doing any activity in which he cannot shine, especially school work, because he is not content to be an ordinary mortal but hopes to become rich and powerful. In the past three years, apparently in contrast with his ambitions, he has, however, started going out with lower-class friends and idealizing Mafia organizations."

A careful decodification of extraverbal messages and of countertransference allowed me to tune in to the mother's states of mind and her feelings during this account: pride ("he is a nice and intelligent boy,") disappointment ("he has started going out with lower-class friends,") and exaltation ("he is idealizing Mafia bosses.") What was already clear at this point was *collusion* between mother and son in idealizing destructive narcissism aimed at feeling powerful (the Mafia bosses.)

Since the mother came to me in order to help her son, I probably placed myself in a suitable position to pick up in transference, and register in countertransference, those aspects of the mother that resembled the son. As I observed and listened to the mother, I wondered if it was she who was identified with the character expelled into the son, or whether it was the son who had a pathological identification with the mother, or if the mother were impersonating the son in order to show him to me "live" as it were. My impression, in any case, was that the son was an integral part of the mother's psychic organization.

EVOLUTION OF THE RELATIONSHIP
FROM OUR FIRST MEETINGS
UNTIL THE START OF ANALYSIS

For a long time Laura did not give me the chance to talk: the sessions were a long monologue, and all I was allowed was some sign of implied assent to express my agreement with points of her discourse that seemed to show some sort of insight. It happened, however, that as soon as Laura realized I wanted to say something, even simply to express agreement, she immediately took back what she was saying. It seemed clear that she tended to establish a narcissistic union with me, in that she did not allow me to emerge as an object other than herself and also that she felt only partially accepted if she felt I agreed with her on only some points, while she expected to be accepted in toto.

All I could do was watch her and listen while she lost herself in a dead-end maze of explanations that were simply hypotheses, clarifications that merely underlined the contradictions, and solutions that were only pseudo-solutions, as well as accept her intense idealization, or, rather, *intense admiration* within a transference that was gradually taking on mirroring characteristics. In order not to lose contact with Laura and with what was happening in the relationship, I tried to avoid the role she had assigned to me of making my tools available for her to use in understanding her son; *her* meaning of understanding was to open his head, to see what was inside and find out what he was thinking and planning to do, rather than what he felt.

In an attempt to introduce the dimension of subjectivity and psychic suffering and to resist her tendency to transform her son into a thing object, I tried to put her in touch with what might be the anxieties and insecurities against which Antonio had built his defenses.

My proposal for her to try to understand her son's suffering from this viewpoint was taken as an invitation to take part in my mental processes, in my functions of linking and reflecting, but it did not lead to any kind of empathy with his deep emotional discomfort. I ran into a similar resistance when I tried to put her directly in touch with her own worries and anxieties abut her son's problems and with the feelings she had when she could not control him. Laura resisted talking about herself and used the entire session to talk about Antonio.

How should the enormous importance the mother gave to her son's problems be interpreted? In terms of the impossibility of her abandoning her fusional relationship with him? As an initial attempt to integrate, in my presence, a split aspect of self, an aspect of self repudiated and expelled into the son? What type of object was the son for the mother? A persecutory introject? An object used as a drug, called upon to play a transitional role and destined to give the subject a sense of being alive and real? (McDougall 1982.) An object containing the mother's bad part and necessary to her narcissistic image? A complementary narcissistic object or "a narcissistically seduced object included in the seductive object"? (Racamier 1992, p. 129.)

Some of the stories Laura told me seemed absurd—for example, that her unemployed son wanted to pay for tutoring with his own money and buy a motorbike with promissory notes—and yet they made me think that Antonio's violent destructive attacks on his parents, perpetrated by constant solicitation and destruction of their love, (Bollas 1989), also contained a desperate and autarchic attempt to get free of the mother's influence; his desire for independence and affirmation of his own identity would be in polar conflict with his desire for fusional belonging. I thought that it was precisely Antonio's extreme *dependency on the mother's mind* that had prevented him from experiencing the pleasure and gratification of being understood and using his own mind in his (suspended) treatment.

Laura framed his problem with drugs and illegal trafficking, about which I was informed at our first consultation, in the form of "a generic doubt about a more or less unfounded suspicion of an anxious mother." I wondered if she was defending herself from something that was very painful and humiliating for her (realizing that her son still took drugs), or whether instead her silence expressed some kind of collusion with him. The second hypothesis, which did not exclude the first, turned out not to be totally unfounded. Laura confessed that for some time she had been giving her son money, without telling Antonio's father ("for fear of his reaction"). Given the clandestine atmosphere in which this was done, it seemed it might be interpreted as an equivalent of incest (Racamier 1992).[1]

In time it became clear that Laura's narcissistic balance and "normotype" rested on two propositions: that it is better to have a delinquent son than a depressed son who is a failure, and that if her son really is delinquent then her worries about his illicit actions and their possible legal consequences are correct perceptions of real facts that Antonio does not want to share so as not to worry her, and not the fruit of her "sick imagination," her "visions," or her "premonitions." Therefore she need not doubt the objectivity and lucidity of her judgment and can consider herself healthy.[2]

---

1. Racamier writes of the "incestuous relations that develop" in psychotic families and in à cloture fermée families generally (families completely locked in a cocoon, refusing any changes) that are "perpetuated without a genital act but through apparently banal and secret acts that are the equivalent of incest, for example, the manipulation of therapists and money exchange" (Racamier 1992, p. 137).

2. E. Jacobson, quoted by Racamier (1980), says that the ultimate aim of any psychotic position is the transfiguration and utilization of objects in

Laura insistently tried to convince me to acknowledge that the situation would ineluctably lead her son to prison or death, yet she showed no trace of concern, the affect which would have been more appropriate to the gravity of the situation. I wondered if perhaps her concern was so great it couldn't be thought, while prison or death represented a solution in that her son would be as yet unborn or would never be born.

The situation of real danger created by Antonio's acting out stirred the whole family. The father, who up to then had been absent, now entered the treatment scene; up to this point through the mother's description, I had been unable to form an opinion about him. The parents also turned to the doctor who had treated Antonio's father for serious health problems in order to discuss their son's problems. The mother asked permission to see me on demand, and I agreed because Laura was clearly unable to sustain the fifteen-day hiatus built into the treatment setting. (My repeated requests to establish a more intensive and regular schedule [once or twice a week] were rejected on the grounds that both she and her son were unable to assume a regular commitment.)

ENTERING ANALYSIS

Laura managed to win a space inside me (and not just in my treatment diary), creating a kind of tension and, at times, a

---

the real world in order to find an external solution to internal conflicts. Hence it is necessary that the real object be a concrete representative, controlled by the subject, of a part of his inner reality. In addition to defensive victory over inner reality, there is supremacy over the object and external reality; they are captured narcissistically. *External reality is therefore considered a narcissistic extension.* Racamier remarks that a real object representing and containing a part of the id is neither more nor less than a successful hallucination.

challenge to find an approach that met her needs and facilitated the arrival of mental representations of her true self (Bollas 1989). I tried to maintain the illusion that I was there, ready to see her, every time she felt like it and to present myself as an object that could be found and used (Winnicott 1968).

I realized that she made personal use of the explanations and indirect comments I offered her concerning what she told me about her son. I use the terms *comments* and *explanations* on purpose because everything formulated as an interpretation not only was ridiculed, but sparked intense persecution and a violent attack against my presumed subjection to Freud. Laura needed to experience me not as an oracle who issued sentences or as a therapist who reasoned with her own patterns, but as a human being equal to her and with whom she could gradually establish a relationship and discover the value of object relations—just as her son, according to her, avoided and criticized hypocritical, bourgeois people in the parents' circle of friends and sought authentic relations with young people from slum neighborhoods.

Breaks in treatment intensified transference phenomena and acting out. Laura began to intuit that her deserting therapy was related to an attempt to control treatment separations. At this point I was able to begin dealing with her directly as a patient coming for herself rather than as a mother coming for advice about her son. However, every direct reference to the infantile self was rejected, while massive projections on her children and the cat maintained constantly active the counter-investment regarding the damaged and avid self. When I tried to put her in touch with the abandoned, excluded, and angry little girl, she answered that she had no such recollection and that she had begun to feel better when she had left home as a teenager, and that her troubles had begun with the birth of her children after a period of being happily married.

By coming regularly to her sessions, albeit still "on demand," and by offering to pay even for missed sessions, she informed me that she was reassessing the proposal of a regular setting, which was now received as an aspect of a reliable and constant maternal holding and as a guarantee against the risk of drug-dependency on an object that can be manipulated and controlled at will. In fact, the drug-addictive nature of the bond with the object seemed to be partially elaborated since Laura thought she was able to tolerate the setting. The session was no longer entirely taken over by her preoccupation with Antonio, and it was clear that her masturbatory insistence on the unsolvable problem of her son coincided with resistance to therapy and her triumphant tendency to annihilate me because I didn't solve her *concrete* problem. At the same time, Laura became aware of her ambivalent feelings towards Antonio and her impulse to free herself of him.[3]

New spaces opened in the relationship and Laura showed me another aspect of her self when she introduced her daughter to me, a brilliant student with many "boyfriend" problems. The day she told me her daughter's psychologist boyfriend had left her because she hadn't wanted to give him the "proof of love," I realized that Laura was very near to giving me this "proof of love" by starting analysis. Three years after our first meeting, Laura began a three-times-a-week analysis.

As a tangible sign of her collaboration she told me her life story, believing this to be what I expected of her since she thought I needed to put together all the details of her life in

---

3. I associate the word "concrete" with the cesarean delivery as a real act, surgically separating mother and child, and I feel the mother's protest to be a preemptory request to help her separate from her son rapidly and painlessly, like a request to mourn, on her behalf, the closure of the birth wound that marked the rupture of the absolute narcissistic union.

order to help her connect with the past in a useful and meaningful way, "above all, useful for Antonio." The more she talked
about herself and her life, starting with her ancestors, the more
her mood improved. She began to rebel against her own
exaggerated dependency on her mother and to differentiate
from her through positive identification with her children who
"are quite rightly angry with controlling and possessive mothers."[4] Her children repeatedly pointed out that she worried
anxiously and counterproductively about everyone and everything, referring to her pessimism, which poisoned the family
atmosphere and induced the various family members to assume
defensive attitudes.

The analytic relationship evolved, in the sense that Laura
gradually became, to use her own words, "more analyzable,"
more receptive, and less frightened of opening up. Although she
withdrew and distanced herself from me each time she projected onto me some archaic persecutory fantasy or when a too
tense emotional contact altered the optimal conditions of temperature, speed, and distance (Meltzer 1976) that favored our
encounter, the experience that anxiety, anguish, and fears could
be contained, transformed, and given meaning through a language shared within *set time limits* reassured her about the fear
that her needs could *never* be met.

In addition to her need for analysis, there was the ego
pleasure linked with feeling that our two minds worked together
on an analytic job. Telling her dreams was an altogether new
experience for Laura. It meant having someone who could
mirror her psychic life and transform the sense elements pro-

---

4. Having to reconcile the two positions of daughter and mother at the
same time puts Laura internally in touch with a "fantasy configuration in
which there is a daughter and a mother who, in turn, is the daughter of a
mother" (Bonaminio et al. 1990, p. 597).

jected on the dream screen into psychic content. In her subjective experience, the dream and the report of the dream were a sign of cooperation in the analysis and an invitation to enter a more intimate and private area of the self and the relationship.

Thanks to the experience of the analytic relationship and the gradual introjection of my "ability to give proper proportions" to situations that seemed hopeless to her, Laura was able, at times when she felt calm, to dominate the violent and contradictory impulses unleashed by, and dumped in, unproductive and exciting arguments with her son. She was also less tempted to use the problem of her son to defend herself or to attack me when she felt frustrated and not understood, which is what happened with her husband.

Working through the relationship with her son was the leitmotif of a long period of Laura's analysis. This is why I referred to *parent* therapy in the title, rather than adult therapy. The more Laura could get in touch with her highly ambivalent feelings towards her son—I stress the ambivalence regarding the "conflict between keeping him in and letting him out"—the more she genuinely wished to understand what failings of hers and her husband's might have caused trauma and deprivation in Antonio. While Laura had wanted to have Antonio, unlike her husband, she felt guilt about having entrusted him to a nanny when he was small, having provided him with gifts instead of attention, and having pestered him about schoolwork. Her reparatory wish to resume the role of affectionate mother, however, shifted very easily into an attempt to control, sustained by an unconscious fantasy of keeping Antonio small and segregated with the excuse that he might get in trouble, just as Antonio was struggling to experience his adolescence and "have a girlfriend like other people his age."

Even her guilt feelings for past errors fed her impulse to exercise control over her son and challenged his right to an independent existence. Indeed, if Antonio went out without asking for money, Laura would be obsessed by the idea that he might meet the wrong kind of company and find the money himself, and if Antonio spent money having fun with rich friends from good families, she felt robbed of her own vitality and lost adolescence. While listening to Laura talk about her son and his problems for entire sessions, I more than once found myself thinking how this son should be in order for his mother to accept him, and I was unable to imagine any way in which he might exist that would placate, sedate, or cure this woman's profound dissatisfaction.

Laura's extremely contradictory account of how Antonio should behave to satisfy her did not help me to find an answer. Her insistence on the disappointment of having a son who had dropped out of school and her repeated statements that she would have preferred a "successful delinquent" suggested to me that the assumption of *a negative identity* by Antonio was not so much—or not only—a rebellion, but rather an adaptive collusive response, coming from a precocious defensive identification with a refusing object (Miller 1986). The fantasy of having a successfully delinquent son seems to have been Laura's sole panacea for the major narcissistic wound of having a failed son, her sole antidote against a deep lack of trust in herself and in her son, not distinct from herself.

It now seemed clear that Antonio's destructive narcissism was induced and sustained by identification with idealized and omnipotent destructive parts of the mother's self that had been projected into him and increasingly took the form of a defense against the mother's depression. Antonio's idleness and failure to finish things, as well as any regressive manifestation, were not only unbearable but triggered hate and rejection when they mirrored and resonated with the sense of emptiness and anxious agitation that Laura compulsively tried to fill by taking in food and pills. Especially in this phase of the analysis the son coincided with Laura's least valued and rejected parts. There also seemed to be a correspondence between *the mistrust of herself, mistrust of her son*, and *mistrust of the analysis*.

I believe that to solve the collusive aspects of the mother–child relationship which subtended and nurtured Antonio's psychopathology, I would have to get a better idea of the position he occupied in the mother's unconscious and of the way in which fantasy projections and projective identifications crossed each other in the mother–child relationship. I will not discuss the details of Laura's family history that might be useful towards exploring the unconscious representations preexistent to her unconscious choice of partner, as well as to the conception and birth of Antonio, and that might confirm the hypothesis that the son's disorder was already inscribed in the mother's unconscious. I will stress, however, that if the mother's unconscious really does gradually emerge during the son's treatment, then the mother's analysis can reveal the aspects of self that the mother splits and projects onto the son and the attitudes and behaviors that the mother induces in him; the gap between the imaginary son and the real one; the internal parental images that the son projects into his real parents (which emerged in Antonio's dreams that the mother shared with me);[5] the fantasies, elements, and contents from the parental unconscious that settle in the child as ego alien factors (Bonaminio et al. 1992, Neri 1993, Winnicott 1969).

I will continue my clinical account of Laura by formulating a series of questions to which I still have not found an answer.

---

5. Referring to Modigliani's theory regarding the treatment of adolescents through their parents, Carbone (1992) maintains that the phantasy projections of the son on the parents can gradually evolve due to real changes in the parents.

When would Laura recognize me as a transference object on which to depend? I still often felt in a position of object exclusion as I believed her husband must have; in fact, for a long time he did not appear in the dream scenario in which Laura saw herself as the sole unchallenged director. When would she let me emerge as a new object? More than once I was told that only her current family was important to her and that she had never had a female friend. Why was the husband absent? Was he too involved in a symbiotic situation with the primary objects or did work substitute for the symbiotic object for him? Couldn't he find space in the mother–child relationship, or did he leave his son hostage to the mother in payment for his freedom? Laura said that her husband was uncommunicative and didn't have any feelings. Why did Laura talk so little about her daughter? Did she represent her functioning part to be kept out of analysis or did she totally identify with her? Could Antonio's symptom be the emerging element of a family pathology?

Laura's contribution to understanding what happened not only between her and me, but also between her family members and herself, oriented my therapeutic strategy in response to her original request: to cure her son.

Since the son's psychopathology should not be seen only in a one-to-one relationship with that of the parents, I tried to correlate it with both their personalities, with the parental couple relationship, and with the structure, functioning, and emotional culture of the family group. Within the family group, Antonio became the receptacle of the damaged self and anxieties and defenses of all the family members. The mother–son relationship seemed to catalyze anxieties about the traumatic and conflictive situations that affected not just the nuclear family but the extended family as well. Antonio's pathological defense organization indicated, as if through a magnifying glass, the narcissistic pathology of a closed family group struggling for survival against annihilation anxieties. These anxieties were projected and controlled in the son through constant challenges to repressive authority and search for support from reassuring figures that functioned as a benevolent superego. The parents' superego pathology appeared in their inability to distinguish between major and minor offenses and between unimportant and important transgressions. All members of the family were drug-dependent (tobacco, alcohol, chocolate), though drug-dependency had socially dangerous proportions only in the case of Antonio.

This extended view of the family's psychopathology is meant to shed light on what prevented the parents from fostering and sustaining the son's treatment once the trauma over the failure of Antonio's earlier therapy had been worked through. In addition to the parents' collusion in sustaining Antonio's narcissistic pathology, which took the form of a blind spot against recognizing his needs and anxieties, a specific *family phantasm* seemed to nurture Antonio's defensive omnipotence: admitting that the son could not make it on his own or with the help of his family would mean for those parents shattering the myth of the family's strength and self-sufficiency, which was incarnate in the male figures of the family.

Working with the mother and not with the family, the only way I could imagine any restructuring of fusional and symbiotic family bonds and redistribution of anxieties was by forming a couple with Laura, a couple that in Meltzer's terms (1986) can perform *the four introjective parental functions* of generating love, sustaining hope, containing suffering, and thinking. Laura's pessimism tended to pollute the sessions, and she doubted the possibility of her son's recovery, based on psychiatric labels without hope. So I offered a solid trusting attitude, which Laura identified in my ability to resist being confused by her tendency to manipulate and destroy me.

Laura gradually shifted the parental couple experience she had in the analytic relationship to her relationship with her husband. She elicited a complementary function in her husband by projecting into him a trustworthy internal object so that Antonio could now become a shared object that both parents looked after. (Antonio had a car accident over the weekend, one of those weekends in which Laura, anticipating the analytical break, escaped with her husband and expelled her needy and rejected self into her son and her analyst. This gave her the opportunity to reflect on the fact that her husband, unlike herself and the analyst, was worried about his son's life and not that he was still out of work.)

The death of one of Antonio's friends in a motorcycle accident sparked small movements towards a depressive position in both the mother and the son. The accident was correctly felt by both as a suicide attack "against the parents." While Antonio mulled over the gesture and commented that Mafia criminals protected each other because they didn't have parents while he had a family,[6] Laura sorrowfully thought that her parents were old and tired and that her husband didn't deserve to be attacked as if he were responsible for everything that happened. I didn't miss this opportunity to put Laura into contact with her son's desire to change and with his sense of impotence and lack of confidence. I had to find a firm but not repressive course of action; in other words, I had to contrast the reality of a just paternal law with the ghost of a bad, sadistic, and persecutory internal penis.

Feeling that both parents were strong and could not be blackmailed, Antonio could begin bringing his real self home

------

6. Antonio began to realize that he owed his life to his parents and that he could count on them, displacing the self-generation phantasm onto the Mafia.

without looking for stand-ins in slum children; he could bring home his angry sense of impotence, his fragility, and the violence and depression triggered by the loss of omnipotence. He tearfully described dangerous things he had done and dangerous things that had happened to him in the past, but the parents could not tell which were real and which were imaginary. Panic, confusion, anxiety over losing himself and "not feeling alive," "of having nothing and being nothing," terror, and hallucinations exploded within the family nucleus. The parents had to contain Antonio's mental states and anxieties and try to give meaning to his apparently mad and senseless behavior. Together with the mother I witnessed the transformation of Antonio's oneiric function: "gradually hallucinations became things of imagination which were then distinguishable from things of reality" (Ferro 1992a, p. 125). Elaborative dreams through which Antonio symbolically communicated specific anxieties replaced the nightmares used to evacuate emotions, anxieties, and monstrous and terrifying images; these dreams were told to me by the mother each time.

I also got an idea of the quality, manner, and functioning of Antonio's inner world from the mother's description of his attitudes, dress, behavior, and the decoration of his room. The presence of internal persecutory objects, archaic object relations, and pathogenic identifications, as well as the fragmentation of the self and poor ego resources, prevented Antonio from entrusting himself to his parents and from separating from them and leaving home. Antonio began to have some important insights: if, on the one hand, they permitted him to see "something he had never seen before," on the other, they set off intolerable anxieties related to areas of nonintegration and the consequent impossibility of assimilating the trauma. The state of fragmentation was aggravated by the activation of the elaborate defense called disintegration (Winnicott 1962).[7] The mother was urging Antonio to go back into analysis, but Antonio refused because he wanted his parents to treat him and "his needs were so great that he would have needed six sessions a week."[8]

The episode of psychotic regression was overcome mainly due to the conjunction of three factors: the containment offered by the family, made possible by my constant attention to modulating the panic, urgency, and violence set off in Laura and her husband by Antonio's regressive behaviors (staying in bed without doing anything, not washing himself, crying); the support of a psychiatrist friend of the family who prescribed a bland psychopharmacological therapy; the support of friends chosen by Antonio himself who represented an "out-of-family hook" to help him accept reality through the re-evaluation of his grandiose fantasies as well as the abandonment of those pathological identifications (Miller 1986) that he so regretted because he "no longer had or was anything."

The situation, which seemed under control, came apart as the result of a life-threatening accident Antonio had. Antonio

---

7. Winnicott, according to Nicolò and Spano (1991), believes that disintegration consists in "an active production of chaos as a defense against non-integration when the maternal support of the ego is lacking, namely, against the unthinkable or archaic anxiety stemming from environmental failure during the stage of absolute dependence. The chaos of disintegration . . . has the advantage of being produced by the child . . . it is in his sphere of omnipotence" (Winnicott 1962, p. 61). Suicide, as an active attempt to defend oneself from liquefying anxieties, may paradoxically become the only affirmation of a self that decides to self-affirm by using extreme methods (Nicolo and Spano 1991, p. 430).

8. I have thought that the title of the present work might have been "history of a disturbed adolescent who set change in motion in the whole family," per Winnicott's perspective on the antisocial trend as an expression of hope containing an element that pushes the environment to become important.

spent the summer vacation with a friend and his family, and it seemed that he had shifted from drugs to alcohol. Back home the parents found a job for Antonio far from the city where they lived, acting out an impulse to get rid of their "inseparable-unbearable son" (Racamier 1992), an impulse that was rationalized in various ways. Antonio's reaction to his parents' acting-out was a serious automobile accident that forced both parents dramatically to acknowledge his extreme fragility and the danger of suicide.

Antonio went into the hospital, where he was detoxified and put on pills. During his long hospitalization period, Laura demonstrated unsuspected energy and organizational abilities for a woman who was normally overcome by laziness, emptiness, and feelings of uselessness. This emergency situation offered her the opportunity to stage an aspect of her self—the director—that had appeared more than once in her dreams, and that permitted her to control her fragmentation and confusion anxieties by coordinating meetings between the various doctors, each of whom was called upon to play the role Laura needed and to impersonate the character she wanted him to assume; in this manner the conflict among several aspects of her self was externalized. The protection offered by the hospital setting allowed Antonio to express in all its dramatic violence his claustrophobic terror and his hatred of his mother and the hospital staff, who he felt were holding him prisoner. At the same time, the parents were able to screen and get to know the friends Antonio wanted to keep in touch with.

Is it possible that Antonio's agitation, anxiety, and terrors, ascribed by the psychiatrist to drug abstinence, could have been due to an extreme vulnerability of his body in the wake of the accident, experienced as a break in his corporal fusion with his mother? If so, then the physical treatment, the consolatory gratification, and the reassurances Antonio received could have offered him the chance to reduce the catastrophic anxieties linked to the experience of being separate and to promote the birth of a feeling of identity. In particular, physiotherapy met Antonio's need to feel strong and male, and fostered the experience of his body as his own and not an extension of his mother's, while adding a new self image that included the sexual body (Laufer and Laufer 1984).

Antonio's return home was a continuation of his convalescence, as both he and his parents continued to satisfy their need for protection and their dependency on nursing staff. When Laura was afraid of dealing with her son's anger, despair, and lack of confidence, she could turn to his father, and derive partial compensation from the presence of a husband of whom she had felt deprived for so many years.

The analysis had been interrupted by the emergency situation but was then resumed. This time Laura reviewed the stages of her life with her husband and focused on her relationship with him and its evolution. After they fell in love and worked side by side on the job, her husband's financial collapse and illness were seen as a serious narcissistic wound. It reinforced the pathological side of Laura's bond with her children by means of a defensive operation that included them in her pathological narcissistic organization (Piovano 1989), equivalent to a narcissistic retreat. The analytic experience opened, or reopened, the path to object relationships. I already mentioned that Laura elicited and acknowledged in her husband a parental role complementary to her own insofar as, in the transference, I became alternately the self and the object and insofar as she discovered me and introjected me as a new protective and transformative object.

The son's psychotic breakdown caused the father to become emotionally involved and perform his parental functions, but it also coincided with the *breakdown of the denial of the father's psychic vulnerability*. It was in this circumstance that Laura discovered hitherto unknown thoughts and feelings in her husband and realized that he was not a machine but a human being who was tired and traumatized by a deprived past. Concern for her husband's health and awareness of time passing urged her to go deeper into understanding the collusion with her children that prevented her from establishing sufficient distance to take on some parental functions and encouraged her turning to her husband only in situations she could not face alone.

The dreams in this period introduced a stage of the analysis "dedicated to the working through of separation from her children." The dreams showed evolution in the sense of relaxing defenses against the wish to know oneself and in the sense of an expansion of what she could think and transform as the result of our meeting. In her dreams Laura prefigured situations of separation from her children so as to try out, in the containing situation of the session, anxieties and conflicts evoked by the telling of the dream (anger, panic, jealousy). The depressive experience connected with separation from her children came out later when the daughter found a job and a boyfriend and when Laura realized that her "unfounded" concern that Antonio might go to jail was an extreme defensive construction against her fear of losing him. The depressive experience of loss and giving up ownership of her children that accompanied the process of mournful divestment of adolescent aspects of the self and led to separation and individuation from her children was modulated and tempered by the recovery of the affective dimension of her relationship with her husband and her parents (facilitated by her experience of an affective quality in the analytic relationship); by satisfaction from having cooperated in her son's therapy like the father of Little Hans (the representation of the self coming close to the ideal self); by greater energy and clarity coming from the introjection of the analyst's parental

functions qua mental functions; and by the sense of psychic
balance she derived from having found a good way to separate
from her children, namely, by creating transitional areas. Laura
was now able to distinguish between the part of herself that
resembled her son and the part of herself she ascribed to her
son, between the real and imaginary son, and between herself
and the pathogenetic aspects of her parents from which she was
now differentiating.[9] Her empathic identification with her children's need to separate gradually from the family actually
functioned as a reparation for her own self, which had been
traumatized by the drastic separations she had effected from her
own parents when she was an adolescent. When her son found
a girlfriend and arranged with his father to start working, I
expected that Laura would overcome a critical moment of fear
that the analysis would end, and would start to use it as "our"
space for finding "a sense of self."

---

9. Badaracco (1992) stresses the importance of de-identification processes from pathogenic parental objects in order to achieve psychic
change.

REFERENCES

Badaracco, J. G. (1992). Psychic change and its clinical evaluation. *International Journal of Psycho-Analysis* 73:209–229.

Balconi, M., and Giannini, G. D. (1987). *Il Disegno e la Psicoanalisi Infantile*. Milano: Cortina.

Baranger, M., and Baranger, W. (1961–1962). *Problemes del Campo Psiconalitico*. Buenos Aires: Kargieman.

Bezoari, M., and Ferro, A. (1991). Percorsi nel campo bipersonale dell'analisi: dal gioco delle parti alla trasformazione di coppia. *Rivista di Psicoanalisi* 37:5–47.

Bion, W. R. (1962). *Learning from Experience*. London: Heinemann.

—— (1963). *Elements of Psychoanalysis*. London: Heineman.

—— (1970). *Attention and Interpretation*. London: Tavistock.

Bleger, J. (1964). Simbiosis: estudio de la parte psicótica de la personalidad. *Revista Uruguay de Psicoanálisis* 6:2–3.

Bollas, C. (1987a). *L'aggressività e l'uso dell'oggetto*. Paper presented at Istituto di Neuropsichiatria Infantile. Università La Sapienza di Roma, June.

———— (1987b). *The Shadow of the Object: Psychoanalysis of the Unthought Known*. London: Free Association Books.

———— (1989). *Forces of Destiny*. London: Free Association Books.

———— (1990). *Origin of the therapeutic alliance*. Paper presented at The British Psycho-Analytical Society, Weekend Conference for English-speaking Members of European Societies: The Treatment Alliance and the Transference. London, October.

Bonaminio, V., Carratelli, T., and Giannotti, A. (1989). Equilibrio e rottura dell'equilibrio nella relazione fra fantasie inconsce dei genitori e sviluppo normale e patologico del bambino. In *Fantasie dei Genitori e Psico-patologia dei Figli*, ed. M. Bertolini, F. Neri, and I. Salseberg-Wittenberg, pp. 67–89. Roma: Borla.

———— (1990). Realtà della relazione e fantasie sulla relazione: l'enigma del rapporto genitori–figli alla luce del trattamento psicoanalitico. *Psichiatria dell'infanzia e dell'adolescenza* 57:595–603.

Bonaminio, V., Di Rienzo, M. A., and Giannotti, A. (1992). *Le fantasie inconsce dei genitori come fattori Ego-alieni nelle identificazioni del bambino: qualche riflessione su identità e falso sè attraverso il materiale clinico dell'analisi infantile*. Paper presented at Incontri Intercentri di Psicoanalisi Infantile of the Italian Psychoanalytical Society, Rome, February.

Burlingham, D. (1932). Child analysis and the mother. *Psychoanalytic Quarterly* 4:69–92.

Burlingham, D., Goldberger, A., and Lussier, A. (1955). Simultaneous analysis of mother and child. *Psychoanalytic Quarterly* 10:165–186.

Carbone, P. (1992). Le radici della mandragola: un trattamento della psicosi tramite i genitori. *Adolescence* 10(2):297–306.

Chasseguet-Smirgel, J. (1985). *Creativity and Perversion*. London: Free Association Books.

Corrao, F. (1986). Il concetto di campo come modello teorico. *Gruppo e funzione analitica* 7:9–21.

Correale, A. (1991). *Il campo Istituzionale*. Roma: Borla.

Del Soldato, G., and Ferrara Mori, G. (1985). La realtà esterna nella teoria e nella clinica di M. Klein. *Rivista di Psicoanalisi* 31(4):551-558.

De Risio, S. (1996). Affetto simbolo e pensiero. In *La vergine del latte*, ed. L. Ancona, E. De Rosa, and E. Fischetti, pp. 85–90. Roma: Cosmopoli.

Di Chiara, G., Bogani, A., and Bravi, G., et al. (1985). Preconcezione e funzione psicoanalitica della mente. *Rivista di Psicoanalisi* 31(3):327–341.

Dicks, M. V. (1967). *Marital Tensions*. London: Routledge & Kegan Paul.

Fè d'Ostiani, E. (1980). An individual approach to psychotherapy with psychotic patients. *Journal of Child Psychotherapy* 6:57–68.

——— (1982). Transformation of anxiety in the relationship between the psychotic child and his mother. *Journal of Child Psychyotherapy* 8:15–23.

——— (1986). *Clinical aspects of ritual*. Unpublished paper.

——— (1987). *Mutismo Elettivo e Psicosi*. Roma: Borla.

Ferro, A. (1987). L'analisi di un bambino come luogo per evidenziare le identificazioni proiettive del terapeuta. *Psichiatria dell'infanzia e della adolescenza*. 54:3–7.

——— (1992a). *La Tecnica nella Psicoanalisi Infantile. Il Bambino e l'Analista: dalla Relazione al Campo Emotivo*. Milano: Cortina.

——— (1992b). Due autori in cerca di personaggi. *Rivista di Psicoanalisi* 38(1):45–91.

Flapan, D., and Neubauer, P. B. (1975). *The Assessment of Early Child Development.* New York: Jason Aronson.

Freud, A. (1945). Indications for child analysis. *Psychoanalytic Study of the Child* 1:127–149. New York: International Universities Press.

Freud, S. (1900). The interpretation of dreams. *Standard Edition* 4–5.

——— (1905). Three essays on the theory of sexuality. *Standard Edition* 7:135–243.

——— (1909). Analysis of a phobia in a five-year-old boy. *Standard Edition* 10:5–49.

——— (1914). On narcissism: an introduction. *Standard Edition* 14:73–102.

——— (1915). The unconscious. *Standard Edition* 14:159–215.

——— (1923). The ego and the id. *Standard Edition* 18:221–232.

——— (1940). The splitting of the ego in the process of defence. *Standard Edition* 23:275–278.

Gaburri, E. (1993). Il senso dell'interpretazione nelle aree cicatriziali psicotiche. In *Psicoanalisi futura,* ed. G. Di Chiara and C. Neri, pp. 79–100. Roma: Borla.

Gaburri, E., and Ferro, A. (1988). Gli sviluppi kleiniani e Bion. In *Trattato di Psicoanalisi,* ed. A. A. Semi, 1:289–381. Milano: Cortina.

Gaddini, E. (1959). *Immagine corporea primaria e periodo fallico: considerazioni sulla genesi dei simboli di forma rotonda.* Paper presented at the meeting "The First Body Image and Object Representation," State University of New York, June, 1961.

——— (1969a). On imitation. *International Journal of Psycho-Analysis* 50:475–484.

——— (1969b). Language and psychoanalysis. Panel on Language and Psychoanalysis (reporter H. Hedelheit). *International Journal of Psycho-Analysis* 57:237–242, 1970.

———— (1975). On "father formation" in early child development. *International Journal of Psycho-Analysis* 57:397–401.

———— (1977). Formazione del padre e scena primaria. *Rivista di Psicoanalisi* 23(2):157–183.

Gediman, H. K. (1989). Conflict and deficit models of psychopathology: a unificatory point of view. In *Self Psychology: Comparisons and Contrasts*, ed. W. Detrick and S. P. Detrick. Hillsdale, NJ: Analytic Press.

Giannakoulas, A. (1983). Immaginazione, illusione, delusione nell'infanzia e nella adolescenza. *Giornale di Neuropsichiatria dell'Età Evolutiva* III(3):331–341.

Giannotti, A., and De Astis, G. (1979). Autismo infantile precoce: considerazioni sulla psicopatologia e sul processo psicoterapeutico. *Neuropsichiatria Infantile* 219/220:943–964.

———— (1981). La patologia del sé nel bambino. *Neuropsichiatria Infantile* 240/241:647–660.

———— (1986). Uso patologico del linguaggio nelle psicosi infantili. In *Il Diseguale. Psicopatologia degli Stati Precoci dello Sviluppo*, pp. 198–208. Roma: Borla.

———— (1989). *Il Diseguale. Psicopatologia degli Stati Precoci dello Sviluppo*. Roma: Borla.

Giannotti, A., De Astis, G., and Natali, P. (1978). Disturbo psicotico del figlio e sua utilizzazione nell'ambito del rapporto psicodinamico della coppia genitoriale. Paper presented at the VIII Congresso Nazionale S.I.N.P. Firenze, October.

Giannotti, A., and Del Pidio, F. (1991). Tra corpo e parola: l'uso del linguaggio come simbolo condiviso. *Psichiatria dell'infanzia e dell'adolescenza* 58:175–186.

Gibeault, A. (1989). Rapport "Destins de la symbolisation." *Revue Francaise de Psychanalyse* 6:1518–1617.

Giovacchini, P. (1986). *Developmental Disorders: The Transitional Space in Mental Breakdown and Creative Integration*. Northvale, NJ: Jason Aronson.

———— (1993a). *Treating Character Disorders*. Northvale, NJ: Jason Aronson.

———— (1993b). *Borderline Patients, the Psychosomatic Focus and the Therapeutic Process*. Northvale, NJ: Jason Aronson.

Green, A. (1973). *L'Enfant de ça Psychanalyse d'un Entretien: la Psychose Blanche*. Paris: Les Editions de Minuit.

———— (1983). *Narcissisme de Vie: Narcissisme de Mort*. Paris: Les Editions de Minuit.

———— (1990). *La Folie Privée. Psychanalise des Cas Limites*. Paris: Editions Gallimard.

Greenacre, P. (1971). *Emotional Growth: Psychoanalytic Studies of the Gifted and a Great Variety of Other Individuals*. New York: International Universities Press.

Grimaldi, S., and Giannotti, A. (1986). La reazione terapeutica negativa. *Psichiatria dell'infanzia e dell'adolescenza* 53:517–526.

Grinberg, L. (1986). *Theoretical and Clinical Aspects of Supervision: The Goals of Psychoanalysis: Identification, Identity and Supervision*. London: Karnac.

Hautmann, G. (1987). Pensiero e sofferenza: il dolore mentale nella situazione analitica e nella clinica. *Rivista di Psicoanalisi* 30(2):197–218.

Hellman, I. (1960). Simultaneous analysis of mother and child. *Psychoanalytic Study of the Child* 15:359–377. New York: International Universities Press.

Jacobson, E. (1964). *The Self and the Object World*. New York: International Universities Press.

Jeammet, P. (1989). Les assises narcissiques de symbolisation. *Revue Francaise de Psychanalyse* 6:1763–1774.

Johnson, A. M., and Szurek, S. (1952). The genesis of antisocial acting out in children and adults. *Psychoanalytic Quarterly* 21:323–348.

Joseph, B. (1989). *Psychic Equilibrium and Psychic Change*. London: Routledge.

Kernberg, O. F. (1975). *Borderline Conditions and Pathological Narcissism.* New York: Jason Aronson.

——— (1980). *Internal World and External Reality.* New York: Jason Aronson.

——— (1984). *Severe Personality Disorders: Psychotherapeutic Strategies.* New Haven, CT: Yale University Press.

Khan, M. (1974). *The Privacy of the Self.* London: Hogarth.

Killingmo, B. (1989). Conflict and deficit: implications for technique. *International Journal of Psycho-Analysis* 70:65–79.

Klein, M. (1929). Personification in the play of children. *International Journal of Psycho-Analysis* 19:193–204.

——— (1930). The importance of symbol-formation in the development of the ego. *International Journal of Psycho-Analysis* 11:24–39.

——— (1932). *The Psychoanalysis of Children.* London: Hogarth.

——— (1935). A contribution to the psychogenesis of manic-depressive states. *International Journal of Psycho-Analysis* 16:145–174.

——— (1940). Mourning and its relation to manic-depressive states. *International Journal of Psycho-Analysis* 21:125–153.

——— (1946). Notes on some schizoid mechanisms. In *Envy and Gratitude and Other Works 1946–1963.* New York: Delacorte Press/Seymour Lawrence.

Kohut, H. (1971). *The Analysis of the Self.* New York: International Universities Press.

——— (1978). *The Search for the Self.* New York: International Universities Press.

Kolanski, H., and Moore, W. T. (1966). Some comments on the simultaneous analysis of a father and his adolescent son. *Psychoanalytic Study of the Child* 21:237–268. New York: International Universities Press.

Lacan, J. (1949). The mirror stage as formative of the function of the I. In *Ecrits: A Selection*, pp. 1–7. London: Tavistock, 1977.

Laing, R. D. (1961). *Self and Others*. London: Tavistock.

Lanza, A. M. (1986). La reazione terapeutica negativa nei bambini psicotici e nelle loro famiglie. *Psichiatria dell'Infanzia e dell'Adolescenza* 53:537–544.

Laufer, M., and Laufer, M. E. (1984). *Adolescence and Developmental Breakdown*. New Haven, CT: Yale University Press.

Lebovici, S. (1988). Fantasmatic interaction and intergenerational transmission. *Infant Mental Health Journal* 6(1):10–19.

Ledoux, M. (1984). *Conceptions psychanalytiques de la psychose infantile*. Paris: Presse Universitaire de France.

Levy, K. (1960). Simultaneous analysis of a mother and her adolescent daughter. *Psychoanalytic Study of the Child* 15:378–391. New York: International Universities Press.

Mahler, M. (1968). *Infantile Psychosis*. New York: International Universities Press.

Mahler, M., Pine, F., and Bergman, A. (1975). *The Psychological Birth of the Human Infant: Symbiosis and Individuation*. New York: Basic Books.

Mancia, M. (1985). *Stati psicosomatici e ipocondriaci: loro relazione con la scissione e la identificazione proiettiva*. Paper presented at Centro milanese di psicoanalisi. Milano, October.

Manfredi, S., and Nissim, L. (1984). Il supervisore al lavoro. *Rivista di Psicoanalisi* 30(4):587–607.

Marion, P. (1993). *Genitorialità e psicoterapia psicoanalitica infantile*. Paper presented at XII Convegno annuale dei corsi di psicoterapia dell'età evolutiva Roma, June.

Masterson, J. F. (1975). The borderline syndrome: the role of the mother in the genesis and psychic structure of the borderline personality. *International Journal of Psycho-Analysis* 56:163–177.

McDougall, J. (1982). *Theatre du Je*. Paris: Gallimard Editions.

Meltzer, D. (1967). *The Psychoanalytic Process*. London: Heinemann.

——— (1973). *Sexual States of Mind*. Perthshire: Clunie.

——— (1976). Temperature and distance as technical dimensions of interpretation. In *Sincerity and Other Works: Collected Papers of D. Meltzer*. London: Karnac.

——— (1985). Folie à deux. In *Quaderni di Psicoterapia Infantile* 12:39–78. Roma: Borla.

——— (1988). *The Apprehension of Beauty: The Role of Aesthetic Conflict in Development, Art and Violence*. Perthshire: Clunie.

Meltzer, D., Bremner, G., Wittemberg, G., et al. (1975). *Exploration in Autism: A Psychoanalytical Study*. Perthshire: Clunie.

Miller, D. (1986). *Attack on the Self: Adolescent Behavioral Disturbances and Their Treatment*. Northvale, NJ: Jason Aronson.

Neri, C. (1993). Campo e fantasie transgenerazionali. *Rivista di Psicoanalisi* 39(1):43–64.

Nicolò, A. (1989). Trauma in adolescenza. *Psichiatria dell'Infanzia e dell'Adolescenza* 56:438–492.

Nicolò, A., and Spano, E. (1991). Regressione nel break-down adolescenziale in corso di trattamento. *Psichiatria dell'-Infanzia e dell'Adolescenza* 58:423–434.

Novelletto, A. (1981). Il sè nell'adolescenza: aspetti normali e patologici. *Neuropsichiatria Infantile* 240/241:595–616.

Novick, J., and Novick, K. K. (1992). The relevance of child and adolescent analytic experience to work with adults. In *Saying Goodbye*, ed. A. G. Schmukler, pp. 285–303. Hillsdale, NJ: Analytic Press.

Pallier, L. (1984). Fusionalità agorà e claustrofobia e processi schizo-paranoidei. *Rivista di Psicoanalisi* 31(3):299–306.

Petrella, F. (1982). La scena della conoscenza nel processo psicoanalitico. *Rivista di Psicoanalisi* 29(1):51–68.

Piovano, B. (1989). Aspetti collusivi nel rapporto tra madre e bambino e tra bambino e genitori rispetto all'area dei disturbi narcisistici. In *Narcisismo Nomos Trasgressione*, ed. S. De Risio and E. Orlandelli, pp. 49–68. Castrovillari: Teda Edizioni.

——— (1991). Valutazione diagnostica ai fini della analizzabilità e intervento psicoterapico breve in ragazzo di 19 anni ricoverato in un reparto psichiatrico negli U.S.A. In *Sublimazione Suggestione, Seduzione*, ed. P. Bria, S. De Risio, and E. Orlandelli, pp. 128–147. Roma: Edizioni Universitarie Romane.

——— (1992a). *The artistic side of personality in a borderline psychotic adolescent*. Paper presented at Third International Congress of the International Society for Adolescent Psychiatry, Chicago, July.

——— (1992b). *Alcune riflessioni sulla funzione del terzo nel processo di formazione dell'identità e di simbolizzazione nelle psicosi infantili*. Paper presented at Incontri Intercentri di Psicoanalisi Infantile, Roma. February.

——— (1996). Simbolizzazione e linguaggio: accesso alla parola nel bambino autistico. In *La vergine del latte*, ed. L. Ancona, L. De Rosa, and C. Fischetti, pp. 182–192. Roma: Cosmopoli.

Racamier, P. C. (1980). *Les schizophrènes*. Paris: Editions Payot.

——— (1990). A propos de l'engrènement. *Gruppo* 6:83–95.

——— (1992). *Le gènie des origines: Psychanalyse et Psychoses*. Paris: Editions Payot.

Robutti, A. (1992). Cassandra: un mito per l'ipocondria. In *L'Esperienza Condivisa: Saggi Sulla Relazione Psicoanali-*

tica, ed. L. Nissim Momigliano and A. Robutti, pp. 195–213. Milano: Cortina.

Rosenfeld, D. (1992). *The Psychotic Aspects of the Personality*. London: Karnac.

Rosenfeld, H. (1987). *Impasse and Interpretation*. London: Tavistock.

Sandler, A. M. (1990). *The treatment alliance and transference in children and adults*. Paper presented at The British Psycho-Analytical Society: Weekend Conference for English-speaking Members of European Societies. London, October.

Sassanelli, G. (1982). *Le Basi Narcisistiche della Personalità*. Torino: Boringhieri.

——— (1987). Narcisismo e strutturazione della personalità. *Rivista di Psicoanalisi* 33(4):495–512.

Searles, H. F. (1986). *My Work with Borderline Patients*. Northvale, NJ: Jason Aronson.

Segal, H. (1957). Notes on symbol formation. In *The Work of Hanna Segal*, pp. 49–64. New York: Jason Aronson, 1981.

Soavi, G. C. (1990). Il mito dell'eterno ritorno e la sua importanza nella ristrutturazione del sè. In *Fusionalità: Scritti di Psicoanalisi Clinica*, ed. G. C. Soavi, R. Tagliacozzo, and C. Neri, pp. 121–129. Roma: Borla.

Tagliacozzo, R. (1982). La pensabilità: una meta della psicoanalisi. In *Itinerari della Psicoanalisi*, ed. G. Di Chiara, pp. 237–248. Torino: Loescher.

Teruel, F. (1966). Considerations for a diagnosis in marital psychotherapy. *British Medicine and Psychology* 39:231–236.

Tolpin, M. (1971). On the beginnings of the cohesive self. *Psychoanalytic Study of the Child* 26:316–352. New Haven, CT: Yale University Press.

Tustin, F. (1972). *Autism and Childhood Psychosis*. London: Hogarth.

——— (1977). *Treatment needs and prospects for the psychogenic psychoses of childhood*. Paper presented at Conferenza sulle psicosi infantili, Università La Sapienza, Roma, October.

——— (1981). *Autistic States in Children*. London: Routledge & Kegan Paul.

——— (1990). *The Protective Shell in Children and Adults*. London: Karnac.

Winnicott, D. W. (1950). Aggression in relation to emotional development. In *Collected Papers: Through Paediatrics to Psycho-Analysis*, pp. 204–210. New York: Basic Books.

——— (1952). Psychoses and child care. In *Collected Papers: Through Paediatrics to Psycho-Analysis* pp. 219–228. New York: Basic Books, 1958.

——— (1954). The depressive position in normal emotional development. In *Collected Papers: Through Paediatrics to Psycho-Analysis*, pp. 262–277. New York: Basic Books.

——— (1958). The capacity to be alone. *International Journal of Psycho-Analysis* 39:416–440.

——— (1962). Ego integration in child development. In *The Maturational Processes and the Facilitating Environment*, pp. 56–63. London: Hogarth, 1965.

——— (1963). Fear of breakdown. In *Psycho-Analytic Explorations*, pp. 87–95. Cambridge, MA: Harvard University Press, 1989.

——— (1968). The use of an object and relating through identification. In *Psycho-Analytic Exploration*, pp. 218–227. Cambridge, MA: Harvard University Press, 1989.

——— (1969). Mother's madness appearing in the clinical material as ego-alien factor. In *Psychoanalytic Explorations*, pp. 375–382. Cambridge, MA: Harvard University Press, 1989.

Zetzel, E., and Meissner, W. W. (1973). *Psichiatria Psicoanalitica*. Torino: Boringhieri.

INDEX

Affective symbolization, encouragement of, child autism, 158–169

Antilibidinal narcissistic structure, pathological collusion, narcissistic disorders, 84

Badaracco, J. G., 198n9
Balcone, M., 167
Baranger, M., 75n4
Baranger, W., 75n4
Bezoari, M., 75n4
Bion, W. R., xviii, 53, 54, 84, 112n5
Bleger, J., 84
Bollas, C., 72, 73n1, 111, 131, 132, 147n7, 181, 184
Bonaminio, V., 109n3, 112n5, 116n9, 139, 186n4, 189
Burlingham, D., 104

Carbone, P., 189n5
Carratelli, T., 109n3
Chasseguet-Smirgel, J., 147, 169
Child autism, 155–171. *See also* Infantile psychosis
cognitive and affective symbolization encouragement, 158–169
identity formation, 155
parental psychopathology, 155–156
symbolizing function of setting, 156–158
third object evolution, 169–170
Child Guidance Center (C.G.C.). *See* Psychopedagogical treatment; Public health service care

ABOUT THE AUTHOR

Barbara Piovano was born in Turin, Italy, graduated from the University of Genoa with an M.D. degree, and later obtained a specialization in child neuropsychiatry. She received her adult analytic training from the Roman section of the Italian Psychoanalytic Society, and has been practicing in Rome for more than twenty years. She is a member of the Italian Psychoanalytic Society (S. P. I.), the International Psychoanalytic Society, the International Society for Adolescent Psychiatry, and the European Association for Adolescent Psychoanalysis. She is Professor of Child Psychiatry at the Chieti University and conducts a child guidance center for children and adolescents in Rome.

Dr. Piovano was awarded a Fulbright Scholarship to attend the adolescent treatment program at the North Western Memorial Hospital in Chicago in 1989 and presented a paper on "The Artistic Side of Personality in a Borderline Psychotic Adolescent" in Chicago in 1992 at the Third International Congress of the International Society for Adolescent Psychiatry. Her paper on "The Collusive Aspects in the Mother–Child and Parent–Child Relationship in the Area of Narcissistic Pathologies" reflects her interest in the reciprocal influence between the parent's mental structure and functioning and that of the child. In "Symbolization and Language Access to Speech in the Autistic Child," she discusses the analyst's function, particularly the notion of the analytic third, in transforming preverbal and presymbolic levels of psychic functioning into feelings and thought that can be verbalized.